THE
SUBTLE
SELF

THE SUBTLE SELF

PERSONAL GROWTH AND SPIRITUAL PRACTICE

JUDITH BLACKSTONE

North Atlantic Books
Berkeley, California

Published by ·
North Atlantic Books
Húichin, unceded Ohlone land
aka Berkeley, California

Cover and book design by Paula Morrison
Printed in Canada

The Subtle Self: Personal Growth and Spiritual Practice is sponsored and published by North Atlantic Books, an educational nonprofit based in the unceded Ohlone land Huichin (*aka* Berkeley, CA) that collaborates with partners to develop cross-cultural perspectives; nurture holistic views of art, science, the humanities, and healing; and seed personal and global transformation by publishing work on the relationship of body, spirit, and nature.

North Atlantic Books' publications are distributed to the US trade and internationally by Penguin Random House Publisher Services. For further information, visit our website at www.northatlanticbooks.com.

Library of Congress Cataloging-in-Publication Data
Blackstone, Judith, 1947–
    The subtle self : personal growth and spiritual practice / Judith Blackstone.
    p. cm.
    ISBN 1-55643-066-3 (pbk)
    ISBN-13: 978-55643-066-4
    1. Self-actualization (Psychology) 2. Movement therapy. 3. Mind and body. 4. Blackstone, Judith, 1947– —Mental health. 5. Dancers—New York (N.Y.)—Biography. I. Title.
BF637.S4B56 1991
158'.1—dc20   91-35756

MQ 24 23 22

This book includes recycled material and material from well-managed forests. North Atlantic Books is committed to the protection of our environment. We print on recycled paper whenever possible and partner with printers who strive to use environmentally responsible practices.

For Zoran,
in memory of our life in the cave.

Acknowledgments

The ideas and methods in this book have been most influenced by the people who allowed me to witness and participate in the mystery of their growth toward wholeness. I offer them my humblest, deepest thanks. I also thank my many teachers, in particular John Daido Loori, Sensei, for his vivid communication of Zen principles and for teaching me Shikan-taza meditation; and Amos Gunsberg for teaching me about the center of the head and the mental dimension of experience beyond the energetic, and for arguing with me until I became a little more articulate in my point of view. I thank Margaret Beals, Daniel and Victoria Rosen, Myotai Treace, David and Debra Draxton, Theresa Delia, and Annette and Oliver Bloodstein for their careful reading of this manuscript and for their encouragement. I thank Jeremy Tarcher for his expert suggestions and Renate Stendhal for her patient coaching and criticism. I thank my husband, Zoran Josipovic, for his understanding that helped me to understand what I was saying, for living with me through the many rotations of this circular vision as it emerged, and for lending me his strength and faith through the painful squeezing of the circle into the linear shape of a book. For the priceless gift I have received from Sathya Sai Baba, any expression of thanks is an understatement. I have tried to thank him in this book by writing with as much integrity as I could about the spiritual reality that he has helped me to glimpse.

Contents

Preface

This book is my personal testimony to the self-healing, self-growing nature of our lives. It is a book about experience, the possibility of refining and deepening what we can know and feel of life.

About eight years ago I emerged from a period of severe physical and emotional pain. An injury to my spine and the subsequent unsuccessful surgery had left me almost immobilized, causing me the loss of a much-loved career as a dancer. My recovery seemed in some sense miraculous because it occurred spontaneously. When I was not helped by conventional means of treatment, I lost hope and retreated into solitude. One day, however, I discovered that by simply relaxing, surrendering to gravity, I could feel an inherent movement in myself toward balance and health. It was a movement of both my mind and my body, a very gradual merging of the two. The merging was accompanied by a sense of coming alive, of moving toward truth. I felt deep contact with myself, as if my mind were awakening in every cell of my body. At the same time, I felt communion with all of life, as if this subtle level of my mind were also the mind of the world, or the universe.

I came back to life transformed, happier than I had ever been, with a deep conviction about the underlying spiritual nature of the universe.

As my injury healed, I studied psychology and many forms of body therapy. I began working as a psychotherapist, meditation and movement teacher. Now I was able to witness in other people the same spontaneous process of growth I felt in myself. Over the years it became clear to me that this process is motivated by a pre-existing potential in us, in much the same way that the seed of a tree is motivated to grow by the powerful vision contained in it. Our potential is wholeness—the total availability of our body, heart and mind to receive and respond to life.

As we grow toward wholeness, our consciousness becomes more subtle. We experience an awakening, a dawning sensitivity to a deeper, more fundamental dimension of life. Here we find an amazing, little-known law of nature: our subtle consciousness is both the innermost core of our individual self and the medium of our communion with all life. In other words, our deepest self-knowledge is also our spirituality, our oneness with life. To fully become ourselves is at the same time to transcend ourselves.

Many of the people who came to work with me had been taught that being spiritual meant shutting down or "outgrowing" some aspect of themselves, such as sexuality, intellect, or the sense of personal uniqueness and initiative. These restrictive beliefs were actually hindering their development. On the contrary, wholeness is an integration, a unity of all aspects of ourselves. If we do not interfere with the process, we grow naturally toward our potential as sexual, emotional, intellectual, spiritual beings.

The following chapters offer an understanding of personal growth in the context of our underlying wholeness and transcendence. I have included many exercises for attuning to the movement toward wholeness both as a felt experience in our body and as the unfolding of circumstances in our lives. I have also described some ways to recognize and release our interference with this movement.

The primary source of my understanding, as I have said, has been my own experience, both healing myself and working with others in what I now call the Subtle Self Work. I therefore begin the book with a brief account of my own story, my inner work, and some of the teachers and teachings that have most influenced me. I believe that we can only speak in a personal voice about the nature of consciousness. But if we fine-tune ourselves to our experience and then communicate with one another, we will gradually come to a shared knowledge and a faith in the unity that infuses our lives with love and meaning.

Introduction

TOUCHING THE EARTH

As a child of eight or nine, I was very attracted to religion. Having once been taken by a friend to the neighborhood synagogue, I afterwards made my way there myself on Saturday mornings. I liked best the atmosphere of concentrated stillness during the silent prayer. I sensed something in this atmosphere that I had not found anywhere else in my life and I wanted to know more about it. But my parents were not religious Jews; my father in particular was afraid that my rational mind would be spoiled by religious ideas. In fact, this book may have its deepest roots in the dialogue that began between us the first time I came home from synagogue convinced that I had found God in the silence, and that God had found me. I was encouraged to go to dancing school on Saturday mornings.

My parents took me to a little dancing school in Sheepshead Bay, Brooklyn, about twenty minutes from our home. My teacher there was a young, intent, dark-eyed woman whose body seemed as taut and impassioned as a forest animal. Her name was Donya Feuer. Although I usually made straight for the shadows in a crowd, Donya's strange intensity of purpose sought me out and beamed into my private little world. I felt chosen and

1

overflowing with treasure. She invited me to do a duet with her, which we rehearsed at the school and performed in 1956 at the Henry Street Playhouse in New York City. There was one aspect of my sudden good fortune which I could not articulate at the time, but which I think made the circumstances more significant for me. The year before I started at the dancing school in Brooklyn, I had a friend who owned a little pale blue gauze tutu, dotted with gold paint, like the costume worn by ballerinas. We spent many afternoons improvising to music in her room, taking turns wearing the tutu. I enjoyed this game immensely, and I often daydreamed that someone would discover me and make me into a professional dancer. It was quite an unlikely fantasy. The fact that it came true so soon and so easily added a resonance, a metaphysical thread to the unfolding of events.

Donya's dance was called "Dust for Sparrows." As she made it and taught it to me, I had the sense that she was looking into my own mute, dreaming mind and giving me the means with which to know myself. One section of that dance I will never forget. I am walking downstage towards the audience with my eyes closed. It is a long walk, about thirty steps, and I must keep very alert, because if I walk too far, I might fall off the stage. So I carefully slide my foot forward along the ground each time before I step. I am imagining that I am outside, walking on earth and soft grass. When I have counted thirty steps, I stop and kneel down, keeping my eyes closed. Then with my right hand, I begin to rub the ground. As I rub, I slowly open my eyes.

This awakening of the senses aptly described my life at that time. The following year, when I was ten, I was asked into the modern dance company which Donya ran with her dance partner, Paul Sanasardo. Although Donya moved to Sweden a few years later, I was to continue to dance with Paul for the next fifteen years. The impact of these two people on my life was both tyranny and inspiration. Capturing my mind at ten, their

work filled and stretched and dominated my imagination. I suddenly had a view of life radically different from the one in my
parents' home. I saw through the artist's eyes a world that was
open to question in all its aspects. I was privy to the confidences
of a group of adults who were engrossed, if not obsessed, with a
search for meaning in a world which they described as absurd
and brutal. Often I would curl up under the table where they
sat smoking Gauloise and drinking black coffee while they
talked, so that I could gather my data on this new world without
distracting them.

As a child performer, I was given mostly dramatic roles,
which initiated me into the study of the psyche. I would have
to "run fearfully" or "jump joyously" or carry various props across
the stage as if portending some ominous or tragic future. To do
this I had to attune myself to my emotional experience, as well
as to my physical body. I became sensitive to the emotional content of gesture both in myself and others, to psychological states
as they register in the body. Although I still went to school and
lived in my parents' home in Brooklyn, my memories of those
years are mostly of this vivid new dimension of life that had
been so abruptly thrust on my unused mind. I sat through hours
of rehearsals, watching the adults dance (later other children
joined the company), as I gripped my prop, getting "in the
mood." I lived in a world of motion. The dancers in the company were the people I was closest to, and what I knew best
about them was the way they moved. Pretty soon I was seeing
everything in my life as a dance. Form, texture, color, sound,
everything was translated by my dancer's mind into vibratory
equivalents, into energies and relationships between energies.
I felt a communion between the aliveness of myself and the
aliveness of this vibrant, dancing world. I had found again the
atmosphere that I had felt in the synagogue, in the stillness
charged with prayer. This communion is still the most satisfying,

most valuable aspect of life for me. As a child and teenager I was willing to go to great lengths for its sake—enduring exhaustion and Paul Sanasardo's increasing domination. In return, I had the rare pleasure of experiencing myself as a finely tuned instrument, capable of expressing the subtle, lyrical dynamism that I sensed in the world.

When I was eleven, it became obvious that I had a fairly pronounced scoliosis (an s-shaped curve in the spine) which made it difficult for me to gain strength. Now I worked doubly hard. By my teens I was taking two or three dance classes a day in addition to rehearsals, and by my twenties I had achieved quite a high level of technical ability. Probably because it took so much concentration to dance with my wobbly spine, I had particularly good balance. I began to receive favorable reviews from the newspaper critics. I was also given ample opportunity to do my own choreography, and the use of our fine dance company. But I was not happy with my work. Somewhere in all the years of hard labor, I had lost track of myself. I had become a puppet, trapped in the character that Paul had seen in me years before and which I played out for him in all his dances. This character, the sensitive, awed child, had at one time been truly me, and then I had needed his recognition to express myself. But gradually it had become a rigid mask which I dared not outgrow. My emotional instability, my need for love, my fear of confrontation had become entangled with my love for dancing. I was no longer growing towards that luminous center I had once sensed but trying desperately to maintain some human contact, some warmth against the flood of confusion and loneliness that I felt in myself. I do not know at what point I began to get lost, but finally I admitted to myself that I was far from where I wanted to be. In 1972, when I was twenty-five, I summoned up all my courage and left the company. I planned to do my own work and form a company of my own.

That summer the choreographer Pina Bausch was coming from Germany to work with us and I stayed on for this last concert. Pina had danced with us when I was a child and I did not want to miss this chance to be with her. Pina had been a child during World War II. Her work reflects the deeply imprinted anguish of her generation. From the first rehearsals, I had to hold a contorted, twisted position which exactly mimicked the distortion in my spine. Although I knew it was hurting me, physical endurance had become an easy thing for me, much easier than giving up. After two weeks of rehearsals, I was in enormous pain. I was so weak that I could not hold a paperback book, and finally I quit.

In retrospect, I see my dance career as a phase of religious development. I had trained myself to give all, body and soul, and it did not matter so much to what: art, love, God. The focus of my life had been dedication, devotion to something outside myself. I had gone as far as I could in this direction and, broken, I was forced into rebound. But at the time I felt terrible shame about my breakdown, and I felt other things too, which I was not yet able to acknowledge: a seething anger at all the people and circumstances that had contributed to my loss of self, and bitter grief for my child's heart that had been too needy and too early exposed in a complex world.

In the next two years, I went to many doctors and chiropractors. I continued to force myself through dance classes; I would pull myself out of pain for a few weeks at a time and then collapse. All the doctors I saw wanted to operate. I was assured that surgery would free me of pain and that I would be able to dance again. In 1974 I agreed to have my spine fused, from the sacrum to the two vertebrae above it, the fourth and fifth lumbar. A slice of bone was taken from my left hip and grafted, like a tree graft, onto the spine, immobilizing that area of my back.

The doctor who performed the operation met me in the post-op room just as I was surfacing from the anesthesia. Bending his head down close to mine, he said, "You have a weird back." The expression on his face was familiar to me—arrogant, impulsive, unseeing. Yet it was also deeply pained, and that too was familiar. It was a face that hurt me and at the same time pulled on me for my compassion. In the slow time of the anesthesia, I felt my conditioned response begin to form; amazed, I watched myself shaping an apology out of the terror and pity that rose in my throat. It was an apology about my whole existence that I had always been ready to feed the compelling, familiar monster who loomed over me now. But this time I did not speak. Exhaustion overwhelmed me, not from the anesthesia, but from all the similar scenes which I had lived through but had only dimly recognized. Now they stood out, stark and unavoidable, in the bare hospital room. This moment marked for me the end of one life, my life of submission and helplessness, focused on the needs of others, and the beginning of another. The doctor's remarkably sadistic comment remains in my mind as the inscription over the entranceway to the underworld which I was about to explore, first as a lost wanderer, and then with increasing skill at finding my way.

Before my injury, I had what is called a "well-compensated" curvature, meaning that my head was centered over my perineum. But during those last rehearsals, I had pushed the curvature out of its balance. Now the doctor had fused my spine in this unbalanced position. I was still in pain, exactly as I had been before the operation, but I could no longer pull myself out of pain (and into alignment) even temporarily. I was stuck, off balance. Having spent the last fifteen years cultivating my sense of balance, this was agony for me. At that time I knew nothing about the body's energy system, but I did know that there was now something strangely static about my whole being. I also had no idea of the connection between the body and the mind, but with my body askew, I felt disoriented. Of course I was deeply grieved at the now certain loss of my dancing, and I was also stripped of the psychological defenses which my agile body and professional achievement had provided for me. But there was more: a new difficulty in thinking clearly which caused me profound anxiety. I also found that I was no longer able to pray; partly out of despair, and partly from the fragmentation caused by the fusion, I could not feel my old connection to God. I was used to being able to look at the sky and sense a communicative presence in the atmosphere, a fatherly presence even, knowing my heart and supporting me in my endeavors. Now this seemed repulsively childish to me, a total fantasy. Whereas I had once been able to fill myself with this numinous presence, my body now felt broken and impenetrable. I was alone with a terrible problem.

Before the operation, I had rented a loft in which to live and make my own dances. Here I lay on the floor every day and cried. I also began a tour of the paramedical profession. I had sessions in Alexander Technique, polarity, shiatsu, acupuncture, rolfing and psychic healing. I took classes in Tai-chi Ch'uan. Someone gave me a book on kundalini yoga and I practiced all the meditation and visualization exercises it described. But always despair would overtake me, and I would return to the supine position on the floor dazed by my misfortune.

It was thus in this position that I first began to notice new sensations in my body. First came the awareness of inner motion. Lying quite still, I could feel vibration all through myself, as well as currents of various densities and patterns. Today I know that many people feel this motion inside their bodies, but the first awakening to it was for me, as it is for most people, an extraordinary event. Although I was hardly moving now, compared to the athletic life I had lived in the past, I was aware of a fluidity I had never known before. I had come upon a new dimension of experience, like putting one's ear to a shell and hearing the sea. This realm could be called the prime, communal revelation of our century in the West: the discovery of energy, the hidden dimension of matter. I had intuited it as a young dancer, but I had not felt it so tangibly in my body. I had often wanted to die since my surgery, but feeling this subtle but unmistakable movement inside myself, this echo of nature's mysterious source, I began to rekindle my love for life.

I began to fast one day a week. At the end of one of these fast days, toward evening, I found myself surrounded by something I had never seen before. The room was filled with a network or web of fine black lines. I went into my dance studio which was almost 1,000 square feet, and that room too was completely filled with black lines. I reached out to touch them and discovered that the same webbing extended out from my hand and arm several feet in all directions. When I moved my arm, the webbing around my arm moved through the webbing of the room, like one delicate pattern passing through another. As I stared at it, I saw that the black lines were shot through with vibrating bright points of fine, white light. I still do not know what causes this webbing, but whenever I see it I feel as if I am looking at the underlying grid, the deep geometrical structure, out of which forms emerge.

I also began to see white and colored light around people and around myself in the mirror. Usually the light around myself was a sick-looking yellow, but if I relaxed I could make it turn green and sometimes blue. And I could see vortices, little spirals of light extending several inches in front of people, and myself, at intervals along the center of the body. Now, when friends came over, they were enveloped in light. These luminous figures would come in, bobbing their spirals, sit down, change color, ask for coffee. I felt a more intimate contact with them, and a kind of reverence (they resembled paintings of saints). Around the same time, I found that I could hear a fine, buzzing sound which seemed to be within and around myself. I felt like I had entered a new realm of existence, and very gradually, my curiosity wore through my grief. Although I still felt that my discomfort was unbearable, I developed a strange optimism about my future. In the cavernous loneliness of my loft it slowly became clear to me that I had only to lie down, to give my small weight to the ground, and rest my mind, and my life would, and in fact was, moving forward. Within me, the little wounded child who had worked so hard in the adult world and finally broken under the strain, said quietly and certainly to herself, in her child's language, "God won't leave me here."

As I became more sensitive, I noticed that there were parts of my body that did not vibrate with the rest, and that the currents of energy would push against those parts like moving water surging against a barrier. I became aware that my pattern of vibration was asymmetrical—there was much more motion on one side of my body than on the other. As this became more apparent, I became more uncomfortable. So I began to experiment with ways to balance myself. I discovered that if I simply mentally located the part of my body that was blocked, vibration would immediately occur in that area and motion would begin to flow through it. I also found that I could mentally locate symmetrical points on either side of my spine or my head (there was a very distinct sensation to symmetry which made it recognizable without doubt), and that holding my attention in this way caused the energy currents to flow symmetrically. When I relaxed my attention, my vibratory pattern would return to its imbalance, but not quite as far; the exercise seemed to set up a kind of bouncing action between the new position and the old. I began to understand that the energy currents were related to consciousness, and that consciousness was the basis of the body-energy-mind system. When consciousness was

9

withdrawn from an area of the body (apparently for psychological reasons, as I will discuss more fully in the following chapters), the energy flow was blocked. This affected the health of the organs and the elasticity of the musculature.

Although I did not stay long with my study of Tai-chi Ch'uan, it taught me some of the most significant information for my recovery. A classic Tai-chi text says that as the energy sinks to the navel, the spirit of vitality rises to the top of the head. One day while practicing I noticed that if I sank my energy downward, there was automatically an upward-flowing energy current. The more I could settle my mind and energy toward the ground, the more buoyant I became. Since then I have found that techniques which consciously direct the energy upward disunify the practitioner and disrupt the spontaneity and cohesiveness of the organism. But if the energy is settled downward, the upward flow happens by itself and the full integrity of the system is maintained.

Another Tai-chi exercise, in which you stand still and imagine that you are hanging from a string connected to the center of your head, was also very helpful. In just reading about it, it might seem as though the string would pull your energy upward, but it is actually an exercise in dropping everything toward the ground. In practicing it, I became aware that gravity does not act on the body, but through the body. And more importantly, I saw that in surrendering to the natural functioning of gravity, my body, energy and mind moved spontaneously toward balance. As I released my own grip on myself, as I relaxed, my spine began to straighten, the muscle spasm around the curvature softened, the energy currents gained power as they became symmetrical, and my consciousness got clearer. I found this to be more meaningful than anything I had ever learned before. Built into nature was the movement toward balance, or symmetry, the movement which could free me from pain. No longer a vague

10

intimation of life moving forward or a child's intuition of a distant God, here was this marvelous, plain fact doing its ordinary job in my ordinary body, as reliable and fathomless as the movement of the planets in space or the rain falling on dry earth.

The process of opening to a more subtle level of experience is really a transformation of consciousness, the basis of all of our experience. It affects everything—our sense of ourselves and all of our senses of the world. I remember that during the first years of this opening, I was most struck by the change in my relationship to space. It was as if I were becoming part of space, rather than a figure in space. The Tibetan Buddhist teacher Trungpa Rinpoche has written that a person is like an empty vase, the space inside being the same as the space outside. I felt as if I were basically empty space and that everything I experienced was an impression passing through this space. I felt actually that I was more and more dissolving into space, and yet I also felt more substantial than I ever had. I had more sense of really existing. Although I had always had a strong sense of myself when I was alone or when I was dancing, I easily lost it out in the world. Particularly after my surgery, when all the familiar outer modes of my identity had ceased, I was very easily "blown away." At that time, I lived near the Bowery in New York City, the street-home of every sort of tragic and deranged person. As I passed them I would feel myself sucked into their various misfortunes and hallucinations, and by the time I reached home, I would feel bruised and shaken up. But as my perception became more subtle, rather than becoming more vulnerable, I became more steady in myself. Being part of space I could allow their wrenching grimaces and voices to pass through me without disturbing me nearly as much. I clearly felt my separateness from them and recognized their transitory status in my awareness. Now I could focus on them if I wanted to. I had the choice of responding to their pain rather than becoming it.

11

In 1974, my ex-husband (we had separated two years earlier) took me to see a video of Trungpa Rinpoche. I had never seen any of the Buddhist teachers and I was fascinated by what I saw as the complexity of his personality. Partially disabled by a car accident, alcoholic, a reputed womanizer, a brilliant and powerful speaker with apparently total faith in the claims of Buddhism, I felt that I had never seen anyone so human. By the time the video was over and he had said that he felt lonelier than a little speck on a landing field for airplanes (in fact, I think this may have been all I really heard of his talk), I was quite interested in learning more about Buddhism.

The next time Trungpa was in New York I went to hear him speak. He came about forty-five minutes later than scheduled, which is the tradition for Tibetan Buddhist teachers. While I was waiting I found myself growing very excited although I was not really sure why. By the time he walked in I was in a state of terrific anticipation, on the edge of my seat with my hands gripping the chair in front of me. Apparently he sensed my intensity, because he looked out over the audience to the back rows where I was sitting and met my gaze. As he did this, I saw something totally outside my sense of reality. His eyes appeared to zoom forward, almost half-way across the auditorium, very quickly, as if carried by beams of light. These vivid, phantom eyes hung in the air for a split-second and then vanished, and he began to speak. This was my first experience of the capabilities of a developed personality. It was a teaching beyond anything he could have said in words. It pushed back the horizon of my own efforts and plans and expectations. This was a world with plenty of room for growing.

I saw Trungpa again several years later. I went to hear a poetry reading given by Trungpa Rinpoche, Allen Ginsberg and William Burroughs. I was again sitting almost in the back of the darkened audience, and I couldn't have been less noticeable to the speakers on the brightly lit stage. I was still quite lost in suffering at this time, uncomfortable in my body and in mourning for my past. But I was enjoying the poetry reading and having a very good time until William Burroughs began to read. Burroughs launched into his usual morbid, symbolic reverie but this time it contained grotesque descriptions of women with disfigured and disproportionate body parts, a catharsis of wounded, vengeful sexual traumata. I was enraged at this portrayal. It was too close to my own self-hatred and representative of an attitude toward women I was already too familiar with. I felt my jaw clench and angry tears veil my eyes. Suddenly I felt Trungpa's presence very strongly, as if he were close by, and I sensed a hand inside the center of my chest. There was nothing sexual about this contact. Very gently and with an intense quality of caring, these fingers prodded around my heart as if unfolding it, as one would fold back the petals of a flower bud. I felt very peaceful and amazed at this strange feat of love. Burroughs continued but I no longer felt like the object of his attack.

I did not see Trungpa again after that, and I never met him personally. He recently died a young, heavy drinker's death. I will never forget the compassion I felt from him.

In 1975, I experienced what I think of as an initiation, a glimpse of a very extraordinary state of consciousness which often seems to happen to beginners, marking their entrance into spiritual work. The 16th Gyalwa Karmapa, the spiritual leader of one of the four lineages (the Kagyu) of Tibetan Buddhist teachers, came to the United States for the first time to perform the Black Crown Ceremony. Apart from hearing Trungpa lecture a few times, I knew very little about Buddhism, but I was steadily growing more curious. My attitude was that of a theater-goer rather than a religious participant. Tibetan Buddhism actually makes very good theater, the sounds and colors and the concentration of the people involved being quite spectacular.

But I remember whatever I saw only vaguely, because I was feeling particularly depressed about myself that day. At the end, I stood in a long line and waited for the Karmapa's blessing, a tap on the head with an object in his hand, and the gift of a piece of red thread. Before I bowed my head for the blessing, I got a glimpse of his large, round, entranced face. He did not seem at all dwarfed by his extravagant, almost wing-shaped headdress, which together with the strangely shaped objects of the ritual suggested a totally exotic or even imaginary time and place. On the contrary, his unwavering dignity, and some quality of balance about him made him seem firmly rooted in the immediate present. By comparison I felt myself to be shadowy and tenuous.

I remember a rainy New York day closing in on this odd event as soon as I had left. Perhaps I had vaguely hoped that the Karmapa would heal me or save me somehow. I returned to my friend's apartment, where I was staying with her cat while she was out of town, feeling that I had exhausted even the most far-out possibilities of recovering my life. I went into my friend's dance studio and sat down cross-legged on the floor. And this is when I finally received the Karmapa's blessing. As soon as I sat down I lost all body consciousness. The room also disappeared and everywhere, extending infinitely in all directions, space was a brocade of brilliant light. Suddenly I was aware of inhaling. My breath filled me with a sensation of bliss, impossible to describe, a kind of orgastic happiness with a much subtler kind of discharge, however, than sexual orgasm. I felt myself rising upward, not in my body, because I felt no body, but in my sense of myself. I was rising and suddenly felt I was going too high up and too fast. I felt frightened. I focused with all my will on a point in space, an exercise I had been practicing from one of my meditation books. This stopped the feeling of moving upward. And then the doorbell rang. I stood up and moved through the thick light toward the door. There was my ex-husband wanting to hear all about the Black Crown Ceremony. Strangely, the fact that he was now translucent with pulsating light did nothing to soften my feelings for him. As he followed me into the apartment, I became intensely irritated at the way he was smiling. I felt that he was playing some kind of benevolent saint, quite out of keeping with my own image of him. It did not occur to me that I might also seem a little peculiar at the moment. Furiously, I sat down at my friend's table and began sifting through the passionate chaos in which she lived. Pantyhose, letters, silverware, dozens of photos of saints and gurus from all over the world spilled out before my heightened but now enraged perception. The picture of an Indian guru caught my eye and gave me a sudden sense of extraordinary depth. He seemed completely natural and at ease, and yet different than anyone I had ever seen before. Although I felt that I wanted to look at the photo for a long time, I could not resist the momentum of my anger. I held the picture up to my ex-husband and said, "You are not a saint. This is what a saint looks like." And then we both looked at the photograph. It was an instant which remains in my memory separate from the fast-moving stream of bitterness that had been the ending of our friendship. It was an instant belonging to that metaphysical thread which, I believe, runs through all our circumstances as the "main plot" of our lives. The Karmapa had given me a vision of myself and my world as a single, radiant loom of energy. In the home of an old friend, another old friend and myself had happened upon the photo of a man who would soon become extremely important in both our lives.

About six months later, my ex-husband came to say good-bye. He was moving out West. By then I had almost ceased going out. I spent the days in my pajamas lying on the floor of my studio, or sitting on the floor chanting, in a kind of autistic desperation, sacred words and incantations I had picked up here

or there. Sometimes I sat huddled in front of the mirror, search-
ing my eyes for some shred of reassurance, for some ember of
the communion that I had long ago felt with myself and the
world. As a child I had been able to pray. I had been able to
line up some point deep within myself with some point far away
and to rest there, feeling complete and full. I had felt a presence
in the sky, the trees, that seemed to answer my own. And this
communion moved in my body, it made me dance. Without
this dance, in my broken body, I could not find my spirit, I could
not find myself. And so I searched the mirror, I did "spiritual
exercises" from books, I lay on the floor and waited.

My ex-husband had not seen me since the day of the Black
Crown Ceremony and he was shocked to find me in such dis-
array. The urgency of my condition touched him and he
confided in me that he had become interested in an Indian
guru. If I wanted, he would go home and return with a picture
for me. I accepted his offer and he came back that afternoon
with the photograph. I immediately recognized Sathya Sai
Baba, the Indian guru whose picture we had found six months
before. He said that I should pray to the picture. He set it up
against some books to make an altar and lit some camphor in a
dish in front of it. The camphor flared with a startling, garish
light. Sensing my growing antagonism to the whole project, he
then said good-bye and quickly left.

When I was alone, I sat with the picture for a long time.
Unlike the first picture I had seen of Sai Baba, this one made
him look bizarrely powerful, almost supernatural and totally foreign, like from some other planet. Pray to a picture? Of a man?
The idea was totally repellent. "You are not God," I accused
him angrily. "A person cannot be God." Then I put my head
down on the table in front of this altar and wept and prayed to
Sai Baba to return God to me, to heal my body and spirit. That
same afternoon I called Air India and inquired about the cost

of going to a place that seemed as far away to me as the moon. A month later, I was on the plane.

* * * * *

India. The discovery of India changed the way I feel about the whole planet. Starving, chaotic, filthy, abrasive with the sounds and smells of over-population and under-education, it is also, and just as shockingly, Bharata, the land of those who love God.

Arriving exhausted at the Bombay airport, reeling from the seventeen-hour flight through space and time, accosted immediately by a smell that is embarrassingly suggestive of undeoderized humanity, collapsed in a cracked plastic chair in the grimly low-tech, sweltering lobby to wait the six hours for my connecting flight to Bangelore, I am astonished to feel a kind of soothing sweetness in the air, a feeling so comforting that it touches some deep, forgotten ache in me to be held and rocked, to be safe and whole. I curl my body around my traveling bag and surrender to the momentum of what now seems an inevitable and familiar journey.

Nine hours later I am in a taxicab, having mustered my most calculating, sophisticated persona to match the cab driver's skill in debating the fare. I am sitting in shock in the back seat as an unimaginable collage of disparate images whizzes by—cows, monkeys, women with clay pots balanced on their heads, factories pouring black, putrid smoke across the road. I hear the relentless shrieking of horns—right of way is apparently won by whoever honks most aggressively. Then suddenly my driver swerves to the side of the road, stops, looks uncertainly at me, and gets out of the car, walking off toward the bushes. I get out too. We are on the edge of a field. I feel what I often feel in the countryside—a fine air going through me, as if the scene enters me, makes me one with it. But never have I

felt a quality this fine or penetrating, almost a voice, which pervades my body, enters my mind, moves in me as my breath. A
voice I have never heard before, coming from far away, speaking
of a reach of life I had never conceived of. I want to run from
that voice, it is too foreign, too powerful, but I know that I can't,
it is part of me, I am made of that fine, vast air. I return to the
cab changed. I have become smaller, younger, a tiny pilgrim on
an immense journey. At the same time, I feel myself almost
growling with apprehension. I do not want to meet this man
who is worshiped as God. I do not want to succumb to India's
entrancing atmosphere. As we careen through the landscape,
even the trees look arched and swooning, too full of air, as if
they would lift off the ground, their roots sliding out of the earth.
I press myself down on my seat, and arrive at the ashram confused, longing, resistant, terrified, ecstatic. From the beginning
I am a rebel. I cannot put the palms of my hands together when
Sai Baba walks out towards his "devotees," I cannot put my forehead to his feet when this great honor is offered me, I refuse to
obey the rule about not hanging out in the bazaar outside the
ashram walls. I hate the hysteria of people pushing each other
out of the way to get the seats closest to where Sai Baba will
walk or sit. Yet I am aware that I am engaged in a subtle dance
of approach toward this strange, extraordinary figure. From the
back lines of his devotees, I watch him intently. I have never
seen anyone like him. He has a quality of thickly packed light,
as if one could pass a hand right through him. His movements
seem perfectly balanced and direct, giving an impression of great
beauty. When he walks, I feel the enormous gravity of his being.
At night I dream that I am disassembling him, removing his
mass of black hair, his face, his arms. I am trying to understand
what he is made of. How is it that someone like this can exist?
What does it mean to my own life? Even as I sleep, I feel my

mind changing, trying to accommodate this new image of human-ness.

And he is approaching me, meeting my gaze, sometimes close by, sometimes across a great distance, with total directness, total accuracy. His eyes are exquisitely expressive, as if his whole being were present in them. Measured against the moments of steady communion with this teacher, I begin to realize that the way I usually look out of my eyes has actually distorted the world I see. I have been seeing with only a small part of myself, a small part of my eyes, that eliminated everything but the ethereal, dance-like quality of the world. Now, as I look more fully, I see qualities I have never noticed before. Form, weight, color, everything becomes more substantial, more real.

In the mornings, I walk up into the hills and try to pray in my old way to the presence in nature. But I still feel cut off, trapped in myself. I am angry at God for the loss of my dancing. Dance was my way of praying, of listening, of celebrating, it was my way of being as beautiful as the life around me. Now I feel hideous, unloved, abandoned. I sit on the rocks and rage moves in me like hot lava. I lie down and sob and I feel a screeching hunger for milk, for some essence to flow from the sky and reach down through my shattered mind and reconnect me to warmth and calm. And very gradually, it happens. The life in the trees and grass and the warm rocks enters my body and joins me to them. One morning, I sit up and see the incandescent trees in silent communion with each other, immersed in love. This is the world, I think, the real world. Whatever happens to me, the world is still this luminous mystery. I will find some other way to celebrate it.

Walking back down the earth and stone path to the ashram, I see Sai Baba speaking to a group of students from a nearby school. Suddenly I see the same communion I had witnessed up in the hills, happening between Sai Baba and the students—

incandescent forms, immersed in love. Now I understand why Baba allows people to call him God. God is in the world as this intimate light, in all forms. We grow translucent, revealing this radiant core of life. The moment I am thinking this, Sai Baba walks toward me. He faces me squarely and smiles. I am peering at an awesome fact of nature, like the myriad galaxies in the cosmos, or the slow molding of a baby in the womb. It is something I have never considered before, such a completed, fully achieved smile. I try to smile back, but the effort hurts my heart, my facial muscles feel rigid, and a familiar taste of shame rises instantly in my throat. And still he smiles at me. I realize that I must face this pain in my heart. I must acknowledge that I cannot return his smile.

During this first visit to India, Sai Baba showed me many displays of his extraordinary abilities. He showed me vivid auras of light around him and astounded me with answers to questions that I had only thought of. Probably the most startling and unbelievable of his abilities is his materializing of objects such as pendants or rings or candy and vibbhuti, a sacred ash used in healing. This he does with a little circular motion of his hand in the air, as untheatrical as one can imagine, and then revealing the object on his upturned palm. At first I wondered whether I was tricked or hypnotized into seeing this. Although I saw him do it many times, I could not believe it for many years and after many visits there. In fact, the way Sai Baba looked and moved and smiled was also as unbelievable for me. Several times I returned home from India to find myself shaking the whole experience out of my mind like some particularly engrossing fantasy.

I have seen Sai Baba do these materializations with his sleeve rolled up, for the benefit of skeptical visitors. I have watched him very closely and each time it was his ease, his total lack of visible effort or showmanship, that made the sudden appearance of the little bit of silver or candy in his hand so remarkable. It seemed so natural that after a while, I became accustomed to it. I began to consider it more strange that we all don't have this ability. But I think that it was not until I had begun to feel and to understand the power of the mind to shape the body, to influence circumstances, that I wholly believed that this gentle, luminous man was actually creating objects out of thin air. He has said that as soon as he pictures the object, it appears. This image of the fundamental creativity of human consciousness was the most important lesson of my work with Sai Baba. In order to know that I could change, and in order to help other people, I needed to see how very far consciousness can develop and how this extreme maturity is reflected in the body. The enlightened man looks different from other people. His mastery is visible, not just in the light around him, but in the coherence of his body. There is a vivid sense of oneness about him, which made it clear to me that fragmentation is what ails the rest of us.

During my second trip to India in 1976, Sai Baba called me in for a private interview. Now I was able to speak to him about my back injury, and the loss of my dancing. "Dance," he said. "Good future is coming." I asked him if I would get well, and he said, "Complete cure. Don't go to any more doctors." Then he leaned a bit closer to me and said, in a more confidential tone, "This is your imagination." "No," I protested, "my spine is fused." "Oh yes, fused," he said. "It is your imagination."

My struggle to get well was far from over, but I believed Sai Baba's assurance that I would, or at least, could get well, and this gave me the courage to keep working. I also felt confirmed in what I had already begun to understand, that the source of my physical predicament was a psychological problem.

The discomfort I felt in my body had a deeper level. It was an emotional discomfort requiring a more inward, finer concentration in order to be reached. I was gradually able to perceive that some of my muscular tension was anger, some was grief, some was fear. These feelings were connected to memories, to real events. They were unexpressed responses that had become lodged in my body. If I attuned myself clearly to the emotional content of my tension, I could recall the events that had caused me pain.

I began the slow, long work of listening to and acknowledging my own story, of developing compassion first for my own losses and thwarted strength, and very gradually for the whole network of circumstances that had troubled me, for the inevitable passing down of suffering and illusion from one generation to another.

In 1977, I trained in the Alexander Technique, a form of bodywork which is partly movement education and partly table work. The Alexander Technique "works on" the student to loosen the joints and align the body. I was an Alexander teacher for a few years, and one of the most important aspects of Alexander Technique came to play a major part in my own work. This is the mental direction of energy.

Energy and, consequently, the physical anatomy, can be directed by the mind, without exerting any voluntary movement. If you tell your back to widen, it will. If you tell it to lengthen, it will. If you tell your heart to beat more slowly, it will, and so on. This insight is crucial to the process of self-healing, although often, in healing illnesses, the psychological causes of the disease must be addressed or else directing your body will be conflicted and not work as well. A related method in the Alexander Technique is to become conscious of the imbalance or tension in the body without trying to adjust it. The mental attunement itself balances the body much more accurately than any muscular manipulation.

Working as an Alexander teacher made it all the more clear to me that the source of most physical tension is psychological and led to me training as a psychologist. I believe that in many ways modern psychotherapy is a form of "religion" superior to the traditional forms. It approaches an understanding of desire and the genesis of suffering far more accurately, and even more compassionately, than that offered in many religious teachings. It takes into account the extreme impressionability of the infant and child, and understands that this confused, wounded child survives in the responses and behaviors of the adult. Therefore, in most therapeutic settings, there is no condemnation of negative feelings and actions. Rather, psychotherapy teaches the attitude of the Buddhist sage Milarepa who, after many unsuccessful attempts to destroy his demons, finally overcame them by inviting them into his room. Contrary to much traditional opinion, life is not that frightening or evil once we know what's really going on, once we understand the root of the greed and hatred operating destructively in the world. In psychotherapy, we are not concerned with either deity or devil. There is only the suffering of the potentially pure heart and the confusion of the potentially clear mind. Therefore, it is not effective to practice either suppression or obedience. It is harmful, in fact, because the good in a person is always subdued along with the bad. What is necessary instead is a therapeutic environment in which one can safely express the full strength of one's rage and the full depth of one's grief, and in this way regain the strength of one's identity and the depth of one's love.

* * * * *

In the summer of 1981, I was living in my loft in Manhattan as if it were a cocoon. By now I was doing with some pleasure the work I had begun in desperation—meditating, chanting, and finding exercises to help me settle deeper within myself, to find the mental basis of my physical body. This healing process was like sand dropping grain by grain through an hour glass. As an Indian poet says, I was adding "a digit of light" to myself every day. Although I still felt uncomfortable, awkward and constricted, when I danced I now felt a buoyancy and fullness I had never known in my life. I no longer mourned for the former image of myself. I had seen past the perimeters of my old life and no longer believed that I had really been happy as that agile, over-extended figure I remembered. But I had not yet found myself in a new way.

With the exception of the people who came to do body-work with me or to take my dance class, and a few very close friends, I had made myself increasingly solitary. I went to restaurants alone, to movies alone, I took trips to the Maine seacoast by myself and came back and sat in my huge empty loft, watching the candlelight, listening, waiting. The city that had always fascinated me now seemed shrill and abrasive. I began to fantasize about moving to the country. I remembered that a friend of mine fifteen years before had mentioned that her mother used to rent a cabin in Woodstock, upstate New York. I chose this little town as the locale of my fantasies. One day I found an ad in a newspaper for the Zen Mountain Monastery in Mt. Tremper, New York, about ten miles up the road from Woodstock. I spent a month there and by the fall I had given up my loft and moved in.

The Zen way of life, in this community, in the mountain countryside, was a dance as grave and exacting as any I had taken part in as a child. I often felt as though I were living in a music box—gongs, bells, wooden clappers, and drums sounding in the same way at the same times every day, as we walked and bowed and knelt and sat with concentrated precision. The first year I felt the repetition steadily penetrating the resistance in my senses, so that sounds and gestures, the smell of incense, the strange message of the Zen sutras we chanted in monotone, all

24

became increasingly clear and vivid. Our long hours of sitting meditation were punctuated by various percussive instruments. At first I felt these sounds beating against my spine, but by the end of the year, I felt them passing through me as if my whole body had become the medium of hearing. Monastic life, although strenuous and in many ways constricting, was a deeply sensual experience for me. I did this dance for fourteen months, and only at the very end of my stay did it begin to seem monotonous, and then even unbearably so.

It was my task to clean the nine altars in the monastery. I had to make flower arrangements for each one with the leaves and wild flowers which grew in profusion on the mountain. With the words of the Heart Sutra, "Form is emptiness, emptiness is form" jostling my brain, I went about the forest and streams, gathering the textures and form and colors of this rich landscape. I felt that I had been deepening a relationship with trees and birds and flowers for thousands of years. I touched the earth and felt the essence of my being quicken and flow in my body.

My job as altar cleaner required that I spend a lot of time alone at the various altars, and in this way I became quite familiar with the Buddha statues throughout the building. What struck me most about the image of this teacher was his lack of pleading. He showed no hint of petition or neediness. The Buddha had reached his enlightenment simply by sitting still, his hands folded and his gaze dropped to the ground. Something in the nature of his own body and mind had allowed him, without any outside intervention, to fully realize his potential for love and clarity. This Eastern concept of our inherent potential for complete enlightenment fascinated me. I wondered what laws of nature could explain the ability for consciousness to unfold unaided. In my own meditation I had been feeling that the more I settled my mind and body to the ground, the more completely the motion of life went through me. The motion itself was bringing me to balance. It was the same sensation I had felt lying on the floor of my loft surrendering to gravity. Becoming conscious of this spontaneous motion strengthened my belief that life proceeds naturally towards enlightenment. It followed that all circumstances, whether painful or pleasurable, should be accepted, should be fully received as necessary elements in this process. There is a Zen koan in which a monk says to the master, "I am looking for the way to Buddhahood," and the master answers, "If you move toward it, you move away from it." We can only discover that we are already on the way.

Chapter One

LEAVING NO TRACE

A General Overview of Personal Evolution

According to Buddhist scripture, the Buddha's first declaration after his enlightenment was that we are each already enlightened. Our actual nature is beyond suffering, he said, but our own confusion obscures it from us.

This means that we do not experience reality, but rather the product of our own imagery, based on misinterpretation, conflicting responses, buried memories. To avoid the pain of this confusion, we progressively turn away from the stimulation of experience. We clamp down on the motion of life itself, which, if unimpeded, would flow toward our enlightened state. In our attempt to save ourselves from pain, we actually squelch our self-healing process, our evolution. The working of our own mind blocks our access to our true nature which is the joy and freedom the Buddha called enlightenment.

This underlying truth, and our distance from it, can be understood like this: it is as if we twisted a balloon—the original shape is inherent in the twisted one, and all tensions, or asymmetries, are a perfect reflection of the balloon's deviation from its normal condition. The twist itself is the path it has to follow to return to its symmetry and wholeness.

27

Oriental tradition teaches that there is a subtle, all-pervasive level of consciousness that never changes, no matter how far askew we twist. A unified intelligence is pushing for expression in its constricted shape. This fundamental wholeness may be what enables us to recognize our alienation from ourselves and to yearn for freedom. Zen expresses it as, "I have never moved from the beginning." The Hindu Vedas call it "the One without a second." As we begin to work ourselves free, we have a feeling not so much of change, but of becoming more what we have always been, or of regaining what we had somehow lost. The extraordinary sensitivity and sensation we gradually attain is actually a realization of the ordinary. We are laying bare what we are in fact most familiar with. The ever-present sense of ourselves we had only dimly perceived, now comes acutely into focus.

In order to describe the condition of an enlightened master, Zen Buddhism uses the phrase "leaving no trace." To understand this, we need to recognize the fluid nature of experience. Life flows. It is a stream of multi-leveled stimulation, passing through the medium of our whole organism. If we were enlightened, that is, if there were no confusion at all in our experience, the moments would pass through us without creating any disturbance in our mind and body. We would have perfect equanimity. Being totally present for, rather than defended against, each situation, stimulation would register and pass, register and pass, "leaving no trace."

Those of us who are not enlightened always interfere in some way with our experience. Either we try to obscure both our perception of and response to painful situations, or we try to hold on, to cling to pleasurable situations. There are many variations of our defensive and manipulative measures. They all have in common that they jar the actuality of the moment by constricting the instrument of our experience—our mind, energy and body. This limitation will further alter the way we perceive and respond to reality in the future. When we defend against the flow of life, the obstructed experience freezes within our organism, leaving its trace on all of our subsequent experience. Thus we gradually twist away from the truth of each situation, away from the natural flow of life toward enlightenment.

Curiously, it is precisely the experiences we wish to reject that remain with us forever, until we acknowledge them. The memories of events we could not bear are lodged in the tissue of our bodies, affecting our personalities and our anatomy, impeding our ability to perceive, feel, think, and act. The cure for this constriction is to reawaken those static moments of our past with our present consciousness, to allow the present to penetrate and flow through the traces of the past.

The basis of our resistance to life is psychological. But because our mind pervades our physical body, our pattern of defense, although basically a distortion of consciousness, expresses itself as a distortion of our entire system.

For example, someone who used to lie in bed at night as a young child, while his parents violently argued in the next room, might grow up with a slight hearing loss. It might not be enough of an impairment to be noticeable, but it would still be less than what would be normal for that person. In order to protect ourselves from what we don't want to hear, we withdraw our consciousness from our ears. When the consciousness is withdrawn, the energy flow in that area is diminished. When the energy flow is diminished, the fascial (connective) tissue surrounding that part of our anatomy tightens and, if held repeatedly, hardens into the physical expression of the defensive pattern.

We are made of a totally interdependent, dynamic unity of parts, and therefore cannot limit one aspect of our functioning without limiting the whole. Obstruction of the energy system in one area impedes the circulation of energy in general. Tension in one area of the anatomy creates imbalance all through the structure.

The location of neurosis in the body as tension and stillness (lack of energy flow) began with Freud's student, Wilhem Reich. This is not to say that the same knowledge did not exist before Reich in Eastern and Western esoteric schools. But, as is happening with a lot of esoteric information today, Reich "rediscovered" it and brought it into the exoteric, professional field as his own discovery, attempting to validate it to his colleagues. Reich claimed that the energy he felt as streamings in the body of an emotionally and sexually healthy person was the same energy he saw as flecks of light in the atmosphere. Reich defended the fact that he could feel and see this energy against a powerful and determined opposition until the last days of his life. The difference between the violent rejection of Reich's ideas in the fifties and the proliferation of mind-energy-body therapeutic techniques in the eighties, marks the dramatic progress our culture has made in understanding the nature of psychological problems.

We can never annihilate our consciousness. We can only bind it. Just as in the image of the balloon, the free mind is still there in the constricted one. Every defensive movement is a binding of consciousness in the body. Most of our defenses become fixed in childhood when we are most impressionable and least able to negotiate our circumstances. Our sensitive body responds like wet clay to the action of the mind.

Wherever we have withdrawn our awareness from our body, such as from the ears in the above example, specific memories of the unwanted experience remain trapped in our organism. These memories are not just images; they preserve the emotional charge of the moment, as well as the quality of the age we were at the time, tingeing our personality and all of our later life with the mentality of that age and with the burden of that emotion. Our choices, responses, and desires as adults all reflect the conflicts and survival tactics of our early years. In this way, the human being grows up to be a bundle of diverse mentalities, varying ages, varying attitudes, and, most confusing for the individual, varying needs. All of this fragmentation lives beneath the surface, so to speak, inaccessible to our conscious integrative ability. Most of us, unless we make some effort to heal ourselves, actually live in the past, reacting to life from this or that twisted-off pocket of ourselves, depending on what the present situation reminds us of.

* * * * *

Our overall pattern of openness and constriction is reproduced in all parts of ourselves, probably even in our cells. This mirroring effect is important to understand if we want to facilitate healing in ourselves and others. In the next chapter, I will describe methods for reading these patterns visually and tactilely, but here is a brief example.

A woman I worked with had been sexually abused as a child. She had withdrawn her consciousness from her pelvis as a defense against fully experiencing the episodes of abuse, and kept her consciousness withdrawn as a defense against fully remembering them. As she approached puberty and began to have sexual feelings, she further divorced her awareness from her pelvis. She wanted to pretend that she was not a sexual being so that she could be sure she would never have to face a situation comparable to the abusive one. The withdrawal of consciousness from her pelvis diminished the energy flow in that area, which in turn caused her pelvic muscles to be tight and hard.

The same woman was greatly encouraged as a child to use her intellectual gifts. Her family were educated, creative people, and always rewarded her efforts in this direction. The ease or

31

openness of her intelligence was expressed in her body as the presence of consciousness, streaming energy and physical health in her forehead and eyes.

We can say that this woman was relatively open in her forehead and relatively closed in her pelvis. If we were to ask her to locate mentally the inside of her forehead area, it would be easy for her to do, her focus would go right to it. But if we asked her to locate the inside of her pelvis, she would have difficulty. Because of the tightened muscles, it would be hard for her mind to get through to that area. If we were to touch this woman's forehead, and if we had developed the sensitivity of touch to detect the flow of energy in the body, we would feel motion, like moving water, beneath our hand. If we touched her pelvis, we would feel stillness, or very little motion.

If we looked closely at the hand of the woman just described, we would see that the bottom of her hand, the wrist, would have less openness, less energy, than her fingertips. The bottom of her hand mirrors the bottom of her torso, her pelvis, and the tops of her fingers mirror the top of her head, the forehead. Hand reflexology and foot reflexology are systems of healing that make direct use of these correspondences. The appropriate areas of the hands or feet are rubbed in order to energize the corresponding parts of the body. The same mirroring effect in the eyes is used for diagnosing illness in a technique called iridology.

Mirroring involves all parts of the body. The wrist alone can be divided into its correspondence with the entire organism; each finger, even each fingernail, is made in the image of one's whole being. As in a hologram, even the smallest part of ourselves is a mirror of the whole. Our personality, our pattern of freedom and inhibition, our unique attitude toward life, pervades us totally, visible in every part of us. This pattern is the shape of our consciousness, our vibrational formation, and it expresses itself in everything we do—in the sound of our voice, the touch of our hand, even the taste of our cooking.

There are many factors involved in our selection of what does or does not affect us in the environment. Little is known about what, at root, makes one person different from another. It is possible that we come into life already patterned by experiences of previous lives, or that there is some astrological imprint on our consciousness at birth. But what we know about the depth of the influence of the parental environment on the development of the child should not be underestimated. Much of our defense pattern is learned in early childhood, and some of it, I believe, is imprinted even earlier. It is likely that from the moment of conception, the new being is subject to his or her triangular relationship with the two general vibratory patterns of the parents. In the womb, and all through childhood, we continue to absorb our parents' patterns of defense and openness. Basic activities, such as eating, walking and conversing, are learned as whole gestalts of vibrational patterning.

Much of the interaction between family members takes place in the more or less obscure ranges of telepathy. A child is molded more deeply by the parents' unvoiced or even unconscious opinions, aversions, aspirations and fears, than by spoken messages which are easier to consider and reject. The general ambiance of the home becomes the air the child breathes; it becomes the shape of the child's breath which later will shape the atmosphere the child lives in when he or she grows up. Some people live with the feeling, for example, that the world is sad, frightening or unpredictable. But what they are responding to is not the world, it is just the traces of their past in their own atmosphere.

The purpose of both spiritual and psychological work is to clear one's atmosphere, to remove the obstruction between ourself and our experience. The master of life, whose experience "leaves no trace," lives in the clear open space of undisturbed awareness, in which the whole of one's life, both one's reception and response, flows uncensored and without distortion. This hypothetical, ideal person is both entirely autonomous and entirely related (without resistance) to the environment, in unity with each moment.

Awakening to unity is the direction and the goal of life. To approach unity, we must fulfill ourselves in two opposite directions, and we are motivated by two opposite primary needs— our need for intimacy and autonomy, for love and detachment. Spiritual evolution is the process of balancing, actually merging, our increasing separateness and sense of self with our also increasing permeability to experience and capability to love. Oneness with oneself is at the same time oneness with the cosmos.

I believe that the process of evolution is life's purpose and its meaning. I am suggesting that it is a spontaneous, natural process which works in everyone in a hidden, muffled way, and in a lucid, direct way in anyone who recognizes and values it. I do not mean to imply that progress is assured, as the accumulation of confusion can outweigh the motion toward wholeness. Hindu teachers say that the mind is like a key in a lock If we turn it one way, it opens, if we turn it the other way, it closes. We are each individually responsible for our own keys, and nobody has the power to turn somebody else's.

But our own vibratory system is inseparable from the vibratory system of nature as a whole. The ever-spinning cosmos produces subtle currents that move through our field of consciousness, impelling us toward balance, toward our essential unity with the cosmos. The movement of gravity moves not on us but through us, pulling us into alignment with the Earth. To resist this natural motion requires great quantities of energy. It is an exhausting struggle which always weakens our physical body.

As we surrender our defenses and open to the motion of the cosmos, our consciousness becomes increasingly refined and expanded. Gradually, this motion penetrates inward toward the core of our body and rises upward through the inner network (the chakras) of the subtle nervous system, giving us access to new realms of sensitivity. (I will describe the chakra system in the last chapter.)

It was Sigmund Freud who discovered an important aspect of the evolutionary process, although he did not think of it in those terms. Freud claimed that our buried life, our repressed memories, the traces of our past, naturally surface. Through dreams, through illness, and through the interesting phenomenon of repetition of similar painful circumstances (he called it "repetition compulsion"), the contents of the unconscious seek admission to our awareness. In terms of evolution, this means that our inherent motion toward completeness, toward our underlying symmetry and balance, involves the release of psychological confusion. Freud said that the principal work of psychotherapy is to help the client release his or her resistance to this surfacing of material. Reality always emerges if we allow it to.

The psychological aspect of evolution is a kind of backward and inward journey. Painful events of our buried past are reenacted again and again throughout our life with new players, until we are able to resolve the pain and confusion of each situation.

The repetition of our childhood conflicts reawakens our repressed feelings, pushing against the rigidities in our body. Loss of love, for example, will automatically touch our grief for love lost in the past, and give us the chance to express and relieve ourselves of the repressed earlier pain. The new oppressive situation will give us the chance to release our anger, to finally stand up for ourselves, and to resolve long held self-images of inferiority and weakness. The process of maturing is to return to our old situations with new consciousness, so that we do not continue to replay our patterns of defense. We can respond anew to childhood dilemmas with the strength of our adulthood, thereby ridding ourselves of old decisions which still affect our lives.

Evolution is thus a partnership between our own effort and the movement of nature, requiring both navigation and surrender. Nature provides us with the situation, but we must apply ourselves to seeing through our own defenses, in order to go on to deeper and subtler awareness.

Amazingly, all of our suffering is nothing but decisions we have made with our own minds to close off parts of ourselves to stimulation. Why have we closed ourselves off from life? As young children, love and recognition are as important for our survival as food. We are extremely resourceful in our determination to flourish, repressing what we know and feel, imitating and adapting to our parents' attitudes, in order to maintain these essential requirements for growth. We fill in with imagery whatever is not available in the environment, fragmenting experience to take in what is nourishing and blot out what is not. None of our decisions are isolated events, but all are made in the context of the dynamic web of psychological economy within ourselves and in relation to the organismic functioning of our childhood family. Every compromise of our own happiness had some necessity, some benefit, which we must now relinquish if we wish to be whole. In order to regain our happiness all that is required is to convince ourselves to change our minds.

Buddha taught that our true nature is obscured by our greed, anger and ignorance. It has been a major contribution of Western psychology to state clearly that emotions constricting life, such as grief, anger, fear and greed, are natural, survival-oriented reactions to the loss, oppression, threat and frustration of our childhood. Deprived of love, we respond to the world with greed; thwarted, we respond with anger; handicapped in all our senses, we can live our whole life ignorant of the abundance which is our birthright. We push and pull and manipulate our already distorted reality, trying to set things right, trying to satisfy our hunger for what is already ours.

The goal of therapy is to help a person become more fully alive, to awaken the blocked currents of life in the body. Our stuck life can be prodded awake by massage or by any method of stimulating and balancing the body. Our conflicting voices can be uncovered and expressed in the psychotherapeutic situation, and our defenses can be shaken loose by stimulating the subtle, central levels of consciousness through a variety of meditation techniques. A lasting change usually requires accurate and specific insights into our past in order to touch and release our actual pockets of bound emotion. We need a thorough understanding of our condition if we are to authentically reverse our earlier decision to constrict ourselves. For deeply ingrained patterns of defense, it can take years of careful reasoning with ourselves to make a difference. I do not believe that maturity can be gained without this specific insight. Knowing oneself is essential for freedom. As our mental level is basic to our emotional (energetic) and physical levels, some people do benefit from purely analytical methods of psychotherapy. But often, repressed emotion is so tightly embedded in the physical structure that effective insight is not even possible. In this case, techniques which directly affect the other levels must be used as well.

However it is done, the process of awakening is the same. It is painful and invigorating. It requires the ability to suffer, the willingness to re-experience the pain of our rejected past while remaining in the neutral, integrating perspective of the present. We are conditioned to believe that pain is always something to be avoided. But anything that has been cramped and numb must hurt as it comes back to life.

It is important, however, not to identify ourselves as this suffering, but rather as the sensation, feeling and awareness that emerge as pain dissolves. The more clearly we begin to experience ourselves, the more we are able to recognize that our old attitudes and problems are only intrusions in our anatomy. They can be dislodged as definitely and methodically as removing a splinter from a finger. While we are learning to respect pain as an aspect of the healing process, we are also learning to desentimentalize it. Pain is only pain, not our identity. It is a sign of where that identity is trying to be born.

Working as a psychotherapist, I hear many people say that they are looking for meaning in life. Most human beings need a feeling of progress, of accomplishment, in order to feel that life is worth living. I know of no greater satisfaction of this need than to progress toward becoming oneself. Christianity uses the phrase "Twice born, once of the mother and once of the spirit," and this does not seem too lofty a description for the experience. As we wake from the spell of our memories, our whole organism is gradually freed. Although this process is very slow and our potential almost infinite, even a tiny step in the direction of wholeness is a great relief. We begin to move more comfortably, our organs get healthier, our senses register a more subtle, more harmonious world, and our understanding becomes more acute. There is an impression of being born to a new dimension of life, both more individual and more vast than previously known.

Whether we use the word God, or mind, or emptiness, or whether we say it is inside or outside of us, it is still beyond us, beyond our immediate knowledge or will. Life passes through us, and the only way to know reality is to open to that passage as completely as possible. It is because of this law of evolution that religion, with its universal teaching of reverence and surrender, has survived the many upheavals in the history of humanity's understanding of itself. We can hold onto nothing as our own. All of our happiness and wit spring from a source beyond our personal ambition. Basically we are each the vessel and the vehicle of the essential motion of evolution.

The mastery of life thus culminates in surrender. Progress is marked by lessons in letting go. But the more we yield to this inevitable stream, the more our life occurs and vanishes without a trace, the more we have a sense of truly existing. We can see with our own eyes, touch with our own hands, make decisions based on our own desires. We regain the vividness of the world and the power of our imagination to dream into being the life we want.

Chapter Two

READING THE BODY

E manuel Swedenborg, the prolific eighteenth-century visionary, wrote, "When a man's acts are discovered to him after death, the angels, whose duty it is to make the search, look into his face, and extend their examination through his entire body, beginning with the fingers of each hand, and thus proceeding through the whole."

If we want to know ourselves, we can make this same search. As I began to explain in the last chapter, our bodies are a record of our psychological history, of both our pain and our happiness. They show the economy of our survival from all the pressures and frustrations of our childhood. They reveal the pattern of openness and defense which makes up our perspective on the world. This pattern is as unique to each of us as the pattern of our thumb print.

Maturity is (ideal) wholeness. Our progress toward maturity, our struggle to regain the lost parts of ourselves, reflects our unique, personal perspective. Psychological theorists have always tried to categorize the various human perspectives, and this can be done to some extent, based on our shared anatomy and needs, and our somewhat common sequence of childhood development and potential difficulties. People fall approximately into distinct types such as the narcissist, the compulsive,

or the antisocial personalities. These divisions are valid and useful, but as is the case with any map, they should never be mis-
taken for the territory itself. The territory is a wilderness and
cannot be truly discovered by anyone but the individual.

The following is an exercise for self-discovery I often give
to people who come to work with me. The experience asked
for may be entirely new for the reader, may seem obscure, or
even impossible. I suggest that instead of puzzling over the directions intellectually, you actually try them. Repeat the directions to yourself "as if" you knew what they meant, and carefully
observe your response in your body and mind. It is really a matter of attunement to what may be an unfamiliar aspect of yourself. If that attunement is not immediately accessible, it might
be by the second or third time you try. The mind sometimes requires several commands before it finds the new "wiring."

Exercise:

Stand barefoot on a level floor with your feet parallel.

Feel the three-dimensional content of your feet. Feel that
you inhabit your feet completely.

Now feel the content of your calves. You are living inside
your calves.

Then proceed to feel the content of your thighs, your
pelvis, your waist, your rib area, your neck and head.

Feel that you fill the inside of each of these areas.

Feel that you are inside your whole body, all at once.

Now return to the feeling of being inside your pelvis. Feel
the space that you inhabit inside your pelvis. Keep focused in
this space and breathe smoothly and evenly. Take note of the
degree of ease with which you can breathe while doing this, as
well as of the intensity and quality of sensation within your
pelvis.

Find the space inside your chest and do the same exercise.
How does the quality of sensation in your chest differ from

the quality in your pelvis? Can you breathe as easily, or more easily?

Find the space inside your head and repeat the exercise again.

Now find the space inside of your pelvis and the inside of your chest at the same time, and keep breathing smoothly and evenly.

Find the inside of your chest and head at the same time, and the inside of your pelvis and head. See if you can find all three areas simultaneously, keeping the breath easy. Take your time with this exercise. The attempt to locate your inner spaces will in itself help to open them, to make them more accessible. Total self-attunement is an ideal.

As you sense the different areas of yourself, be aware of any images or feelings or memories which occur to you. Try not to push away this mental or emotional content, but instead settle into it, really experience it. As you allow it to enter your awareness fully, you will be able to penetrate beyond it, to settle more deeply into your body.

One woman with whom I did this exercise was able to feel the space inside of herself everywhere but in her pelvis and throat. My own observation matched her self-diagnosis. Her pelvis and throat seemed more dense and still than the rest of her body. When she tried to rest her attention in those areas, her breath became labored and her expression changed to that of a young child, about four years old. I asked her to settle her mind into her pelvis as best she could, and to tell me if she could feel any particular emotion. Yes, she said, she could feel fear. She thought it was strange that she had not been aware of this fear before. I asked her how old she felt when she focused on the fear in her pelvis. She said she felt around four or five. Saying this, she suddenly felt pain in her throat, and put her hand there as if to stop the upsurge of grief. I asked her to try to settle deeper into her feelings of grief and fear and to see if she could tell me what was happening around her, or who she was with. "I just think of my father," she said. "I see him staring at me." At this her face contracted with pain. "It seems sexual," she said. For the first time since I had met her, her anguish did not seem restricted to her face, but seemed to issue from her throat and her chest. Although it seemed like a tragic moment for this sobbing woman, her arms wrapped tightly around herself and her whole body trembling, I could see that the pain tearing loose in her was freeing her from the bonds that had limited her life for many years.

Later she was able to detect that she tightened her pelvis automatically whenever she thought of her father. This was her protective stance toward him. It was accompanied by a tightening in her throat against the pain of losing a man she not only feared but also loved. She also realized that she tightened herself whenever any man looked at her. She was able to gain direct insight into how her childhood response to her father had shaped her way of experiencing life. Although she wanted very much to have a relationship with a man, her unconscious fear had been literally shutting out the exchange of sexual energy with the men she met.

Through purely analytical psychotherapy, this woman might have discovered that the quality of her father's attention had often frightened her, and that she now projected the same threat onto other men. But without understanding how that fear affected her body, without experiencing that she was actually holding fear in her pelvis and that she was chronically tightened against the reception of male sexual energy, she might never have been able to dissolve her pattern of defense and overcome her fear.

People usually come to therapy to resolve some current problem in their life. It is sometimes difficult for them to see the relationship between their present situation and their attitudes toward life, formed long ago in their early childhood. The therapist speaks from a frame of reference which they may never have considered, and seems to perceive things about them of which they themselves are unaware. Self-diagnostic exercises, like the one I just described, can be helpful to people at the beginning of therapy, to discover for themselves the validity of psychotherapeutic theories. Further, they can begin to develop the capacity for insight right from the start, so that they have neither to accept nor flatly reject the suggestions of the therapist.

Another woman who was able to use this mind-body exercise to understand herself was Jenny, who came to me because her marriage seemed on the verge of breaking up. She wanted to know what she could do to prevent this catastrophe. She came to me because as a therapist I was supposed to be able to correct life problems much like a dentist can correct tooth problems. She told me that she had been away visiting relatives for about a month. Since her return home, she had felt little affection for her husband. She felt bored by his conversation and even repelled by his physical touch. As we talked further, she acknowledged that she had felt this way somewhat for many years but not as acutely as she did now. She was afraid that she could no longer bear it. Listening to her, I began to feel that her concern was not so much for her own unhappiness. She feared her husband might sense that something was amiss and become angry with her. When I suggested this, she readily agreed. What could she do, she asked, to set things right before this happened? But when I tried to probe her fear of her husband's anger or her dissatisfaction with him, I came up against a very firm, blank wall.

I told her that she would understand the difficulties in her marriage better if she understood herself better. I began to ask her questions about her childhood and her relationship with her parents. But Jenny assured me that there had been no problems in her childhood home. In fact, she had very few memories of her life before her adolescence, and they seemed to her perfectly ordinary and benign. I spent several weeks with her, trying to touch the childhood roots of her unhappiness. But having come to therapy to avoid enraging her husband, she was not about to risk disloyalty to her parents as well, even in fantasy.

One day I asked her to stand up in the middle of the room to do an exercise. Jenny was a tall, vivacious woman with honey blonde hair and warm blue eyes. When we sat talking to each other, she liked to lean forward toward me as if to weave me in or encircle me in her story. Now as she stood up and moved away from our two chairs, I felt for the first time the intensity of her loneliness and her fear of this new journey toward her own self. She stood and looked across the room at me. A muffled flash of anger appeared and quickly vanished in her deep eyes. Standing ten feet away from me, she could no longer feel the bond that we had built between us. I asked her to try to make contact with herself, to really feel like Jenny. "How do I do that?" she asked. "Put your attention inside your chest, try to find a familiar feeling in there, something you've felt all your life." Timidly she probed inward, looking for some sense of herself. Suddenly her whole body seemed pervaded with sadness. I asked her if she could feel this sadness. She said, "I feel a black sphere around me. It is very still." When she said this, I too became aware of an intense stillness around her. I asked her if she could tell how old she was when she first had this sphere of stillness around her. I watched her trying out different ages as she thought her way back into her past, and finally she said that the earliest she could feel it was about three years old. Then I asked if she could tell what was outside the sphere. Again I watched as a three year old Jenny, as still as a cornered animal, probed very cautiously the atmosphere around her. As she did this, the sadness in her body deepened to anguish. "My parents are fighting, they're really screaming at each other. I can't do anything to stop them." She put her hands over her ears as if to blank out the long forgotten sound. She sobbed, first like a young child calling for help, and then like a grown woman grieving for a terrible loss. This was the beginning of Jenny's exploration of her past. She had glimpsed the continuity of herself, and she had felt the open, anguished heart of her childhood. Now she could finally remember how she had closed herself off from her parents' angry atmosphere. She had thought of herself as a social, extroverted person, but she actually maintained at all times a protective stillness around herself which prevented the intimacy she wanted. She also understood her tremendous fear of conflict, and how that had kept her from confronting the problems in her marriage.

Jenny's "black sphere" is another example of the way we defend ourselves from painful stimulation (e.g., our parents' fighting or our father's sexual stare) and then retain this defense throughout our adult life. Each of our defenses relates to some specific (usually repetitive) circumstance in our past. To release a defense, we need to come fully into contact with the memory we have defended ourselves against. This is a process of literally coming to our senses. When we allow ourselves to see, hear, feel, and understand our painful memories, our senses are free to function clearly in the present.

It is important to appreciate the tenacity of our defenses, because it shows us the strength of our own mind. Our "opponent," whom we must reason and grapple with over and over, is the mind of our own child self whom we know intimately and for whom, once we recognize him or her, we can only have compassion. This child's mind is not at all separate from our own present mind. With practice, we can attune ourselves to the child's mind held in our body. We can become fully conscious of our childhood will which is defending our body against experience.

Emily was a young woman who chronically contracted her forehead and temples. Although her head was actually narrow at the top, as if in the grip of some kind of vise, she had no sense of the fact that she was "squeezing" her head. It was not until I began to work the muscles free through deep massage that she began to feel the tension there, but she was not able to let go of it. She was not able to feel that the holding was something she was doing—she felt that the tension was gripping her.

We can say that this long-held contraction was unconscious. But it had not always been unconscious. When I asked Emily to grip her head actively, she remembered that it had been dangerous in her family to be too conspicuous. As a small child she used to try to feel smaller, and thus safer, by contracting the top of her head. Over time, this defense had become habitual so that every time she felt threatened she would automatically contract her head. This way the tension had finally become chronic, and her muscles had lost their flexibility and remained in the defended position.

To massage muscles back into flexibility is an easy thing to do, but it is not enough. The tension will return unless we release the command to the taut muscles. To do that, we have to experience that we are making that command. In order to locate and attune ourselves to the command, it is helpful to know at what age and under what circumstances the defense had first been organized.

* * * * *

We can more easily contact the hidden part of ourselves if we understand the subtle interplay between awareness, emotion and sensation. These levels of experience can be described as vibrational fields which interpenetrate one another. We never have a thought that does not have a component of emotion and sensation, we never have a sensation that does not contain an element of emotion and awareness, and we never have an emotion without the presence of sensation and awareness. The more integrated we are, the more we will have some amount of sensation, emotion and awareness in every part of our body, although the emphasis will differ in each area.

Although never appearing in isolation, the levels of awareness, emotion and sensation can be singled out as distinct qualities, emanating from specific parts of the body. We can fine-tune ourselves to perceive these qualities. If, for example, we tell ourselves to locate our level of awareness, it means to tune in to the awareness already present in us. We are already aware of ourselves and our environment. This awareness has a light, fine, mirror-like quality. To locate our level of awareness means becoming more aware, not just of ourselves and our environment, but of the awareness itself which reflects this information. If we close our eyes, we can no longer see the environment, but that fine, reflective quality is still extended in space. It pervades both the inside and outside of us. If we sense the level of awareness very carefully, we may be able to discern that it emanates from the center of our head.

If we tell ourselves to become aware of our emotional level, this again is an attunement to a particular level of our experience already present in us. It has a slightly heavier, more organ-like or hormonal quality than our level of awareness. It emanates from the chest area. For many people the level of emotion is the most difficult to locate. As our emotional level is often laden with old grief or anger or anxiety, we may avoid contact with it. However, there is no moment of our lives which does not have some emotional content. Life becomes flat and meaningless if we are not open in this dimension. People with little emotional contact sometimes complain that life doesn't feel real, or that they don't feel really engaged in it. As they do become aware of this level, the emotional residue of the past dissolves, and they gain a general feeling of well being and an easy flow of fresh responses to life.

The third level we can attune to is sensation. Sensation emanates from the pelvis area. It is our kinesthetic sense through which we orient ourselves in space. Our level of sensation delineates our physical boundaries, it "grounds" us in our separate, individual self. It is also the level through which we are able to perceive the quality of sensation in other people and to recognize the different textures in the environment. In fact all three levels of our experience allow us to "read" the corresponding level in other people.

Just as there is no method, no "how to" for remembering a scene from our past, there is no way to explain how to attune to these levels, but we all possess this ability. As I said earlier, the best way to go about it is to give yourself the command, as if you knew how to do it, and then watch yourself for the appropriate response.

Find your level of awareness.

Find your emotional level.

Find your level of sensation.

When these levels are fairly clear and distinct, try to attune to any two levels at the same time, always keeping your breath smooth and even. Then try to find all three at once. Be very patient with this exercise Although balance is our optimal condition, it is an ideal, and a life's work at the least. Each of us lives more in one level than the others, but we are all capable, eventually, of opening our attention to our full spectrum of consciousness.

Another way of locating the different levels of ourselves is the adjustment of our visual focus. As I explained in the last chapter, the pattern of our consciousness (where we are open and where we are blocked) is reflected in every part of our bodies.

It affects the way we look out of our eyes, which in turn, affects what we see and how we interpret what we see. People who are most attuned to their level of awareness will look primarily out of the upper portion of their eyes. This is usually the gaze of the intellectual, or, a little higher, the visionary. Primarily emotional people will look out of the center of their eyes, and people who are based mostly in sensation will look out of the lower portion of their eyes. (Many of our sexy movie stars utilize this type of gaze.)

If you find a point on the wall at eye level, and relax, and breathe, you may be able to shift your focus. You may feel how this changes the placement of consciousness in your body, and how it relates to the three levels I have been describing.

Look at the wall from the upper portion of your eyes.

Look at the wall from the center of your eyes.

Look at the wall from the lower portion of your eyes.

Can you recognize your characteristic gaze?

The more contact we have with our whole selves the more we see with our whole eyes. This gives us a much more complete and multi-dimensional view of life. From our whole selves we see a world of meaning, of spirit, of feeling, of texture and form.

The eyes have been called the mirrors of the soul. Whatever transpires in the vibrational field of a human being is reflected immediately and vividly in the sensitive transparency of the eyes. Although the same information registers all through the body, we can easily see, looking at a person's eyes, how they feel at the moment, and how, in general, they look out at the world. We recognize our kindred spirits by looking into each other's eyes. We know instinctively when we see eye to eye with someone, and we know how to negotiate with our eyes the pathways of reciprocal experience.

As we "see through," we penetrate our psycho-physical defenses, and come to inhabit our bodies more fully. This is reflected most visibly in the depth or shallowness of the eyes. Although looking into the body may be an unfamiliar experience for many people, most of us know what it means to look into someone's eyes. We may be aware that some people have a flattened, shallow gaze. When we look at them we seem to be looking only at the exterior surface of their eyes, while with others we seem to be able to look deeply into them. There is a kind of permeability to these deeper eyes allowing our own gaze to enter into and beyond the surface.

I sometimes suggest to people I work with that they look into their own eyes in the mirror once in a while, so that they can witness the visual "proof" of their deepening contact with themselves. In medieval Japan there was a monastery of Zen nuns who practiced "mirror meditation." They would sit in motionless meditation in front of a looking glass, with the intention of sitting until they saw the Buddha.

Actually the whole body has the same potential permeability as the eyes, and is the same sort of gauge of a person's consciousness. As we evolve, the body becomes more subtle. As we gain consciousness in the depths of ourselves, the body deepens, just like the eyes. The more contact we have with our whole selves, the more the various levels of ourselves (sensation, emotion, awareness) integrate. With this integration, the physical body becomes increasingly permeated with the receptive, expressive and expansive properties of the mind. We become conscious of ourselves through the whole substance of our bodies. Wherever we are conscious of ourselves, another person's consciousness can also penetrate. In the same way we look into another person's eyes, we can look into a person's body.

It is said that the bodies of people who are extremely evolved are so subtle and so at one with the mind that they are no longer bound by the usual limitations of matter. The famous Hindu guru Paramahansa Yogananda gave several examples in his Autobiography of a Yogi of occasions when he saw advanced yogic masters pass through walls or levitate to the ceiling. This is not "astral" travel, in which part of our consciousness apparently separates from the body and passes freely through matter, but the physical body itself in its most integrated state. Although most of us are far from this mastery, even a tiny advance in consciousness changes the quality of the body.

All of our senses are capable of becoming sensitive enough to read the mental and energetic levels of another body. With attunement to ourselves, we also become attuned to others. We can feel what it is like to be in another's body, to sense where they are open and where they are defended. Ida Rolf, the woman who invented the deep muscle bodywork referred to as "Rolfing," is said to have had this ability to a high degree. She was able to feel what was going on in the bodies of the people her students were working on, even from across the room with her back to them.

All thoughts, feelings and sensations are alterations in our vibrational field, and these changes are perceptible in the same ways as our more general pattern of openness and defense. By vibrational field I mean the combined interplay of the levels of awareness, emotion and sensation which underlies our body and extends beyond it.

Visually, the vibrational field can be perceived as light, or as motion. Just as we can detect the life force in a flower or a tree as vibrancy, the less defended areas of our body will look more alive, more present, than the other areas. The radiance of the vibrational field has been called the aura. But the aura is often described as only the light around the body. I am speaking about the whole substance of the body as light and vibration. Both the quality and the expanse of this light changes as we become more open, and it also changes from moment to moment with all of our responses. The sensitive eye can look right through the body of another person, through this permeable vibrational field. Actually, many people can do this once they become aware of the possibility. Like the self-attunement exercises I described, it may take a few tries before you find the right focus for this unfamiliar task.

When we look through another person's body, we usually see that some areas are easier to look through than others. They seem deeper. The more shallow areas are denser; the eye cannot as easily penetrate them. However, focusing on the denser areas, we may detect the particular quality which is bound in the tissues of the body there. What looks at first simply like tension may, in a sense, begin to speak to us; we may understand its long-held message. The quality of sadness will look different than the quality of anger or fear. We may also see the quality of a particular age: the grief of a four-year-old looks different than, for example, the grief of an eight-year-old. The rage of a six-month-old infant looks different, even held in the body of a forty-year-old adult, than the rage of a three-year-old child.

We can have the same experience when we touch someone. When we touch a body that is healthy and open, we feel its aliveness as depth and warmth and as multiple levels of vibratory motion. Wilhem Reich referred to this motion as streamings because that is how it feels, like moving water. Just as when we visually perceive depth or shallowness, the less defended areas of the body will seem deeper to the touch. Our own warmth and sensation of touching seems to penetrate all the way through the body, whereas the defended areas are more difficult to contact. They receive our touch only superficially.

Buddhist teachers refer to the individual as a "continuum" of experience over time. Interwoven with our physical body is the memory body of all our past ages. We can locate specific points in this continuum in the same way that we attune ourselves to different levels of our consciousness. Sitting here, I can imagine that I am twenty years old, and instantly feel my sense of myself at that age. I recall my sense of my body, my general emotional state, even the tenor of my younger mind. I feel both the boldness and the timorous excitement of that age, and my pained confusion at being newly adrift in a vast, unknown adult world. I feel the way I hold my body, with my chin a little too high, and I feel the comfortable dreaminess of my imagination. Now I tune a little further back in my memory and remember myself at fifteen. My sense of myself is different at this age. My emotional tone is more intense, with greater contrasts of courage and loneliness. My confusion is dense around my head, and I sense a dark jungle of images from the anguished literature and knotty philosophy I was absorbing at that time. I also feel a bright, giddy sexuality which wells up in me as a new, insistent presence. And further, I can take myself back to my tenth year, my fifth year, my sixth month, even into the womb, recalling the feel and sense of my existence. Any point in our continuum is available to us. We can return with our adult abilities of reason and compassion and address the old pain and confusion which still burden our present-day consciousness.

Recently there has been increasing interest in psychological problems originating in the first few years of life. Those problems are hard to pinpoint because of the non-verbal, pre-cognitive nature of our very early experience. Even if they are not severe, they leave us with a pervasive, ungraspable undertone of loss or defiance or helplessness, an inexpressible sense of something not quite right. It is important that we bring our consciousness to these deep, early levels of memory if we want to deepen our contact with ourselves.

I worked with a woman named Miriam for several years who had complained from the start that she had difficulty concentrating. She would get inspired ideas for creative projects and then be unable to focus long enough to follow through with them. Miriam had a history of childhood abuse which she remembered vividly. Several of her older brothers had repeatedly sexually molested her over a period of many years. She had worked hard to salvage her ability to value herself and to love others from the fear and loathing that this abuse had caused her. But she still felt that her lack of concentration limited her chances for a fulfilling life.

One day one of her brothers admitted to her that he had molested her when she was an infant of five or six months. She came to her session with me badly shaken and almost disoriented. I had not seen her look so vulnerable since we had first met. Having had years of experience recalling her childhood in therapy, her brother's confession was all she needed to find herself as that six-month-old baby. Although she could not remember the incidents themselves, she again felt the terror and intense confusion she had suffered at that age. She felt as if she could not contain herself, as if she were bursting into fragments. As I held her hand to reinforce her link with present-day reality, she allowed herself to settle slowly into the sensation of that terrible confusion. With this settling, she was able to touch a depth of herself she had never reached before. At first she grasped my hand tightly, feeling an overwhelming disorientation, the response to abuse by someone too young to make any sense of it at all. Then the confusion began to disperse and she rested in this new depth of herself. Having reached beyond the confusion, she came to a sense of integration which was in itself the concentration she had been seeking.

* * * * *

A person is integrated when there is optimal interaction between all the vibratory levels of his or her organism. This means that, without adjustment, one is aware of one's entire being all at once. The lack of fragmentation between the various parts of ourselves is what is known as wholeness. We can only reach our fundamental sense of joy and clarity, compassion and creativity, to the extent that there is balance and fluidity in our vibrational field.

Buddhist writing says that our natural, undefended condition is both being and knowing, inseparably united. If our organism is unfragmented, it means that we know ourselves, that we are cognizant of ourselves throughout our entire organism. This state of unobstructed self-knowledge expresses itself in the body as grace and smoothness (like a rock smoothed by the sea), and as an intensity which can be seen and felt by a sensitive observer.

In the past ten years we have seen an increasing number of teachers from the East working in America, and many of these teachers have been living illustrations of the concepts they teach. We can tell that people are wise when we see the depth and strength of their gaze, when we feel the warmth and subtlety of their energy, when our own hearts open in their presence.

Zen Buddhism has many references in its literature to the tangible effects of psychological development, and the recognition of the unified mind. One Zen story has the Master Joshu visiting two hermits in their mountain retreats. At the first hut he asked, "Anybody in? Anybody in?" The hermit thrust up his fist. Joshu said, "The water is too shallow for a ship to anchor." At the second hut he also asked, "Anybody in? Anybody in?" That hermit thrust up his fist, too. Joshu made a profound bow. What could Joshu tell from the two gestures? He could tell that the hermit was very much home, by his bodily movement: the depth of the individual expresses itself in the depth of the body and the way it moves.

Zen students are always asked by their teachers to show their degree of enlightenment, never to describe it. There are many exchanges in Zen literature in which the student asks the master, or the master asks the student something like, "What is Buddha-nature?" or "What is the Way?" The other answers with a shout or a gesture which contains the full measure of the person.

Each religion (and each culture) develops a different kind of depth, largely because each focuses on a different aspect of the body-mind, either directly in its practices or through the emphasis of its teachings. For example, Zen students are taught to focus on a point below the navel, which is the center of gravity for the physical body. The Hindus usually focus on the heart or between the eyebrows at a point called the "third eye." These physically embodied centers are all gateways to the core of life, but each produces different qualities of personality and different orientations toward life in those who work with them. Since presently just about any form of practice is available, some people may find it helpful to choose among religious teachings as a whole, using whatever seems most relevant to their growth at the time.

I think that in our time the teaching and practice of body work and psychotherapy should ideally be learned together with spiritual practice. In any effective therapeutic situation, the emphasis is on the unfolding of the person's individual process of maturing. It seems easier in this situation to remember that we are trying to realize ourselves and not the pre-existent ideals of a particular tradition. Unless we understand our own and other people's motivations, our relationship to the world and to ourselves will always be somewhat obscure and defensive. Our senses become clear when we know our own selves, intimately and specifically.

Chapter Three

THE METAPHYSICS OF SPACE

Unified Consciousness

Zen Buddhism tells a whimsical story about a Chinese master called Tao-Sheng who lived in the early part of the fifth century. Buddhism was still young in China and Tao-Sheng's assertion that all forms of nature had Buddha-nature was not accepted by his contemporaries. But the master was so sure of his intuition that he went out into the desert and discoursed on this subject to the rocks. The rocks, the story goes, nodded to him in agreement.

Consciousness is everywhere, in every atom and every cell. It is the basic element in nature which encompasses and permeates all others. It is the vast space within and beyond all of our experience, out of which everything, including our ordinary mind and ordinary space emerges.

Personal evolution is a growing communion with this fundamental, unified ground of life. It is literally an expansion of our personal consciousness in space. As we gain access to subtle levels of consciousness, we experience them as degrees and qualities of spaciousness, as changes in our relationship to space.

We feel that space is passing through the substance of our body. We have a sense of permeability, or clear-throughness. Our senses (Buddhism counts cognition as a sixth sense) become synchronized until it seems that we have only one sense, one constantly changing, multi-dimensional vivid impression of both inner and outer space, inner and outer life. The Tibetan Buddhists describe this unified consciousness as "the open dimension of the total field of events and meanings."* They say that it has the qualities of clarity and bliss. Christ described it as "making the eye single." The Gospel of St. Matthew (6:22) reads, "The light of the body is the eye: if therefore thine eye be single, thy whole body shall be full of light."

The fundamental level of consciousness is always with us. We are all capable of some amount of attunement to it. Here is an exercise for this "single-eyed" consciousness:

Close your eyes and become conscious of the space inside your body.

Keeping your eyes closed, become conscious of the space outside your body.

Now see if you can feel that the space inside yourself and the space outside yourself is the same continuous space.

Now open your eyes and repeat the same exercise.

This may be easier to feel in some parts of your body than in others. We are more open to life, to space, in some areas of ourselves. Here is another exercise for understanding what is meant by openness to space:

Move your hand slowly back and forth, about five inches each way. See if you can feel that space is passing through your hand as you pass your hand through space.

---

*Lipman, K., Norbu, N., *Primordial Experience* (Boston: Shambala Publications, 1987).

The Hindus call the fundamental level of consciousness Brahman and they say that it has three attributes: sat, chit, ananda—truth, intelligence, bliss.

These qualities—truth, intelligence and bliss—are ours at the core of our being. We do not experience them because we have constricted ourselves in our defense against painful stimulation. Each of us, being open and closed to life in different ways, has a uniquely limited shape and size of spatial consciousness and therefore a uniquely limited reception and response to the world.

Love and Detachment

Interestingly, our bound consciousness is an entanglement of ourselves and the environment both psychologically and spatially. Take, for example, a woman who has had a troubled relationship with her mother. When she was a child her mother's love was not forthcoming in a consistent, wholesome way. Therefore, she closed her heart against her feelings of disappointment and abandonment. She did this by tightening the deep muscles in her chest.

Psychologically, she is entangled by projecting her memory of her rejecting mother onto other women. She both yearns for them and pushes them away. Spatially the contracted muscles in her chest constrict her experience of life in general (constricting her body-mind), thus limiting her personal space. She has lost perspective, both psychologically and spatially.

Our bound life always haunts us. Our painful memories, below the surface of awareness, always project their shadow across our reality, forcing us to create circumstance after circumstance to fulfill our unvoiced, unconscious needs. "I will not let you go until you bless me," we say to our parents, our lovers, our children. Needing them, we cannot love them. Craving their recognition, we cannot see them. Lost in memories, we mistake our present situations for the earlier ones which we have not yet been able to leave behind, responding again and again in our old way.

The Indian poet Kabir called love and detachment the "twin streams" of enlightenment. Detachment is not an unfeeling state but a great resilience to stimulation, and therefore necessary for our full responsiveness, for love. To dissolve our defenses against life means to resolve our entanglement with life. We are able to let life in, really, when we can accept it as it is, when we no longer manipulate or distort it with needs and images from the past. Becoming detached from our projections frees us to witness ourselves and others on increasingly subtle levels without clinging to or rejecting what we see. Detachment does not mean turning away from the world. The motion of turning away is precisely what entangles us.

Love and detachment are twin streams because they grow simultaneously. The more deeply we are able to let life in, the more deeply we are situated in ourselves. We begin to live in the center of our space, where we are most autonomous, where our individuality completes itself. The resolution of the self-environment entanglement is the self-environment unity, the "total field of events and meanings," and at the same time, the full measure of our individuality.

The fundamental ground of life has no center, it exists everywhere uniformly, but we perceive this ground by opening to it through the subtle channel along the central axis of our body. Becoming "centered" is literally becoming conscious in this subtle, integrating channel in the central core of our body. Along this channel are the vortices or "chakras" which, when stimulated, emanate the full potency of our sensation, love, intelligence and spirituality.

Our central axis is blocked from our consciousness by the densities of bound life in our body. As we allow life to pass through us and touch this core, our perception of space expands. The sense of division between ourselves and our environment dissolves as we grow inward toward our core. Physically, as well as psychologically, objects and people seem further away and yet more vivid. This is our true perspective.

Here is another exercise for becoming aware of space:

Begin by sensing the space in front of you.

Now sense the space behind you.

Sense the space in front and behind you with equal attention. In other words, balance your awareness of the space in front and behind you.

Sense the space to the right and to the left of you, and then sense both at once with equal awareness.

Do the same with the space below and above you.

Try to feel that you are encompassed in a 360 degree sphere of awareness with equal awareness in all directions.

You may notice that when you feel space in two opposite directions equally, you also automatically feel the space in the center of yourself. The attainment of balance requires, and is, the attainment of centeredness.

As we gain accurate distance from the people in our lives, we are not only able to love them, we are able to witness their pain without panicking. Having, at least to some extent, become one with that unwavering ground of consciousness, we know that even the most terrible loss or trauma cannot damage people fundamentally. There is a level of ourselves which cannot be broken, cannot be molested, cannot be lost.

Beyond Suffering

I worked with a forty-five year old woman who had been repeatedly raped in her childhood. Every weekend her unsuspecting parents would drop her off at the home of an uncle who would rape her. When I met her she felt damaged irrevocably. Like most victims of childhood abuse, she felt a deep and overwhelming sense of shame and self-hatred. She had blocked out much of her memory of those weekends, and in the beginning of therapy any recollection was accompanied by severe nausea and almost unbearable images of filth and humiliation.

But even those memories could not tear her apart. She gradually came to realize that they were only memories, embedded in the underlying strata of pure, unchanging consciousness. Eventually she was able to allow herself to feel again the terror of her childhood as a sensation moving through the steady field of her being. She had gained a deeper perspective; she recognized the terror as belonging to her past, and she recognized herself as existing on a more fundamental level than that of any passing circumstance, no matter how painful.

A young man reported to me that he was afraid to look in another person's eyes. His mother had been bitterly unhappy when he was young, and he grew up acutely sensitive to pain in the eyes of other people. He always reacted by feeling pain himself, as he had with his mother. But as he became more centered in himself, he was able to see beyond the pain in others to the causes of their pain and further beyond to their potential for happiness. The Tibetan Buddhist teacher, Trungpa Rinpoche, said that compassion is seeing through confusion. Beneath all of our confusion is that dimension that has "never moved from the beginning." Our existence is deeper and vaster than both our suffering and our memory of suffering.

The following is an exercise to help people feel the fundamental stability and permeability of the unified ground of consciousness. It is most helpful for sensitive people who have difficulty feeling separate from the thoughts and feelings of people around them. It is an exercise in letting outside stimuli pass through the clear space of one's field of consciousness. When we defend against life, we limit our own experience. If we can let life pass through our consciousness, we can live fully and spontaneously without feeling endangered or overwhelmed.

I first ask the person to attune to his or her field of consciousness in its full spectrum of awareness, emotion and sensation. I then say that I have a sweet, red candy ball in my hand, about the size of a cherry, and I show the person the imaginary ball. I then throw the ball gently through the person's field of consciousness, first through the space above the shoulders, and then through the person's body. This tossing motion is not entirely imaginary. Pretending to toss the ball produces an actual energy force in the space. Many people flinch or subtly close their field of consciousness against this force. This exercise is practiced until the defensive motion does not take place.

Growing attentive and open to the stimuli passing through our space, we learn to distinguish our own field of consciousness from painful or abrasive elements in the environment. Of course we will still respond emotionally to the other people in our life, but we will not unwittingly "take on" the feelings of others, mistaking them for our own. Nor will we feel the need to limit our consciousness as a protection from such feelings.

Relationships in Unified Consciousness

We can know nothing of the world except what comes to us through our senses and intuition. The quality of our senses determines the characteristics of the world we perceive. Certain aspects of nature, such as the light emitted by a tree, will be entirely lost to us unless our vision is refined enough to detect it. For this reason, our experience of the world is shaped by our particular design of openness to life, or, as we have seen, to space.

Science has discovered that the solidity of matter which most of us experience is not its true nature. All matter is made up of rapidly spinning patterns of energy in vast space. As we evolve, that is as we ourselves become more permeable, the basic fluidity of the world is more apparent.

In this sense, it can be said that we each live in a different world, depending on our own fluidity or density (defendedness), our own personal space. We each relate differently to our world as well. A more fluid world is easier to influence. If I know that the body is not simply a physical mass but also an organization of vibration and consciousness, it is easier for me to change certain conditions of it. Many people have, for example, cured themselves of severe illness using visualization techniques. What would be a hopeless illness or a desperate situation for one person is more easily corrected for another. But at bottom, these differences between people are simply a matter of perspective. Although we each cloak reality with our own painful dream, we all dream in relation to the same center. The steady light of truth, intelligence and bliss at the core of each of us provides, innately, a standard for human values and a direction toward a common goal.

It is because we all live, in fact, in the same basic space (with more or less fluidity) that relationships are possible. The most subtle, pervasive dimension of space-consciousness is our basis of communion with everything in the universe, since everything we can experience has emerged, has crystallized from this source. As we become more open, the communication between us becomes more fluid, or complete, and the sensation of our meeting more pleasurable. We become aware that our exchange is actually a passing through of one vibrational field with another. This is what the Hindu gurus mean when they say, "you and I are the same one," and why Hindu philosophy teaches that we are all different forms of one person. We are each a modification of the same unified space.

The excitement of our meeting with one another, our "passing through" one another, stimulates the release of our defenses. Zen teaching describes a "mind to mind transmission" from the master to the student. Consistent contact with a person whose mind is balanced and open has a balancing effect on our own mind. The master's degree of spaciousness, of unified consciousness, expands the spaciousness of the student's mind.

The basic affinity among human beings extends toward everything in nature. We are able to resonate with plants and animals and even mineral life, because all forms are created by the same laws, out of the same spectrum of vibration. Although human beings are far more developed in the subtle ranges of intelligence, we are actually designed according to the same polarity of heaven and earth which exists more or less obviously in all forms of life. As we become conscious of the full breadth of our vibrational system, we find that, like the Zen master confiding to the stones, we can speak the language of anything in nature. We can feel the love and the mentality of animals and plants, and understand something of their experience. We can find our own foundation, our actual relationship to the earth, by attuning ourselves to the sensation of rootedness in plants and trees.

When the boundaries between subject and object dissolve, we sense a stillness or emptiness in our minds. In this clear space, life imprints itself without hindrance. We *become* our experience. The poet Rainer Maria Rilke describes this unification of the senses when he writes in his Sonnets to Orpheus, "You have created a tree in the ear." He thanks Orpheus, the master musician, for creating forms out of vibrations that can be heard at the same time as they are seen.

Consciousness and Matter

I am proposing that the experience of consciousness as space is the link between subjective, psychological reality and the physical universe. I believe that an integration of Buddhist and Hindu viewpoints with the discoveries of modern physics can produce a coherent model in which consciousness is seen as the ground of all life.

Buddhism speaks from the viewpoint of personal experience about the workings of the mind. To my knowledge, Buddhist teachers never assert that mind and space are the same, but they do say that the experience of pure mind is like clear space. They also say that this space-like experience, sometimes called "emptiness" (Sanskrit: *shunyata*), is not a vacuum, but rather a dynamic openness and potentiality out of which all other experiences arise.

Hinduism speaks from a more metaphysical perspective in terms of the workings of the universe. Hindu metaphysics maintains that mind arises from God (Brahman), energy arises from mind, and matter arises from energy. Each level is considered to be a contraction, or condensation, of the level it arose from. They say that everything in nature is made up of a combination of these levels, and the density of any form is determined by whether its particular formula falls more toward matter or more toward mind. In other words, all phenomena are made up of varying degrees of contraction of God. God is described as the *sat, chit, ananda* at the core of all life.

As I explained in chapter two, the subtler levels (God and mind) pervade the denser, and thus are the integrating ground of the universe. The subtler levels are more expansive and also more stable and enduring than the denser levels. Hinduism teaches that the physical world is only a tiny ripple on the vast ocean of energy and mind from which it emerges. The relative durability of mind provides them with a plausible basis for their belief in the survival of a body of memories and psychological tendencies through successive lifetimes.

Albert Einstein described the identity of matter and energy in his famous equation: $E=MC^2$. In his General Theory of Relativity he also proved that matter is a condensation, or concentration, of space. He spent the last years of his life attempting to prove mathematically that all the basic forces of nature (electromagnetic, strong and weak nuclear energy, and gravity) are transformations of one unified field—space.

I think it is possible to view the eastern and Western pieces as belonging to a single puzzle. Together they form a concept of a wholistic universe in which consciousness and matter are stages of a continuum. All physical as well as psychological phenomena are transformations of the vast space which is also consciousness. The physical space that Einstein studied is itself a transformation, a contraction, of the underlying space of unified consciousness. Therefore, as we become more attuned to our most subtle dimension of consciousness, we become increasingly unified with the ground of all life, with the cosmos itself. This is why it is said that the highly evolved spiritual master is omniscient and omnipresent. If consciousness and matter are stages of a continuum, of one multi-layered vibrational field, we can consider that both these aspects of life are governed by the same laws of motion, such as gravity and inertia, and we can view personal evolution as the natural result of these cosmic laws. Every form in the universe is a contraction, or density, of the ultimate space of unified consciousness. We ourselves are each a particular contraction of space, but our destiny is to expand toward ultimate space, our ultimate reality.

The Direction of Evolution

The idea that all life is suffering, which is called the first noble truth in Buddhism, can be interpreted on different levels. On the surface it means that everything is transient, that we must all know loss and old age and death. But I think that more deeply, we can say that nature itself is the product of conflict, that without the discomfort of imbalance, there would be no life. Complete enlightenment, the end of suffering, is the resolution of this very conflict which gives us life, which drives us forward. According to both Hindu and Buddhist understanding, complete enlightenment marks the end of the round of birth and death for the individual soul, the end of embodiment. The process of opening to life is simultaneously the process of becoming free of life.

Everything that lives must suffer the tension of its incompleteness. Yet as that tension is released and we grow toward the balance that is (ultimately) our undoing, our life becomes increasingly rich with our essential qualities of clarity and bliss.

Eastern religions teach that the path to enlightenment is the dissolution of the ego. By ego they mean everything we do to obstruct the flow of life. This teaching is often misunderstood, or presented in a confusing way. We don't become less as we dissolve our ego. On the contrary, for the long duration of our relative existence, the sense of self intensifies. As long as our individual consciousness is growing toward completion, we are growing toward our center, becoming increasingly balanced, integrated, and secure around our center. That center is the clear, unobstructed sensation, emotion and awareness of being that emanates (or is attuned to through) the core of our body. It is the full measure of our humanness. Very few people have ever totally realized this potential, but it is the direction of evolution.

As we become more integrated, the sense of "I" takes on an unmistakable fullness and cohesiveness. According to Hindu philosophy, this "I" which expresses itself in the deepest currents of our experience is the same "I" which emerges in everyone. As we grow toward our own center, we grow (very gradually) toward the basic identity of the whole, toward *satchitananda*.

But that center is not a blank, impersonal state; it cannot be reached by disassociation from our personal experience. Rather it is the most thorough contact we can have with ourselves. It can only be reached by allowing ourselves to live our own actual experience, which has a unique shape and perspective, and is a unique path for each of us. There is great personal strength and self-esteem, as well as pleasure, in becoming real. We become more autonomous, more separate, as we learn to let life pass through us. We arrive at the calm of genuine privacy—the ability to be alone in our body without shutting off awareness of the environment, without shutting off love. I am emphasizing this because so much of mass religious teaching tends to discourage the full development of selfhood. By admonishing us to suppress aspects of our nature, such as our sexuality or our inquiring mind, and by shaming us into putting the needs of others before our own, such teachings badly stifle our growth toward wholeness.

It may be, as some of the Eastern teachings suggest, that perfect symmetry, or wholeness, is never reached by the individual human being. Sai Baba writes: "Freedom is independence from externals. One who is in need of the help of another person, thing or condition is a slave. Therefore perfect freedom is not given to any man on Earth, because the very meaning of mortal life is relationship with and dependence on another. The lesser the number of wants, the greater the freedom. Hence perfect freedom is absolute desirelessness."

The physicist Heinz Pagels, in *The Cosmic Code*, says, "From the view of modern physics, the entire world can be seen as the manipulation of a broken symmetry. If the symmetries of nature were actually perfect, we would not exist." From this perspective, we can view the incomplete human being as an expression of that broken symmetry. And the path toward perfection is the approach toward symmetry. An important aspect of this path is that we release our manipulation of our true nature, our underlying wholeness.

The broken symmetries of the universe create the tension and the polarization of qualities we recognize as space and time. Perfect symmetry exists (at least hypothetically) beyond space and time. All the polarities that make up the dynamics of our lives move toward integration as we evolve.

Polarities are actually contractions of continuums. For example, the body-mind dichotomy is a contraction of the underlying body-mind continuum, or spectrum. We experience the mind as separate from the body because we have defensively withdrawn our consciousness from our body. As we release our defenses, we realize that there is nowhere we can definitively draw the line between physical and mental experience. Because polarity is conflict and contraction, resolution is experienced as expansion. In this example of the body-mind dichotomy, both our physical and mental experience become richer as the dichotomy is resolved.

Another example is the duality between the intuitive and analytical aspects of the mind. Most of us approach problems more with one half of our mental faculties than with the other. The result is a distorted, limited understanding of the world. As our mind balances and expands, however, we can use all our faculties at once.

As we have seen from the above examples, enlightenment (perfect balance) consists of resolving conflicts between various polarities. It is a process of disentanglement in which each of our functions becomes more complete as they reach a condition of merging. The major polarity for the individual is between inner and outer space, between subject and object. As we begin to sense the continuity between inner and outer space, between subject and object, we also develop a continuity of awareness, feeling and sensation within our own bodies. We have a sense of inhabiting ourselves completely, and we are aware of our whole body all at once. We are able to feel and think at the same time. Intuition and reason support each other. Life is at once actual and symbolic. The maturing intelligence discovers that the world is round, or almost round, and that life is a mandala in which all of the parts become more distinct and meaningful in the context of the whole.

The more balanced we become, the more attuned we are to our fundamental consciousness. And as we approach access to the unbroken ground of ourselves, all of our senses become more acute to the detection of balance. We find that we have an attunement to balance in pitch and in form and color and taste. (You may notice, if you repeat the exercise for balancing your awareness of space, that both your vision and your hearing become clearer.) When I lived at the Zen monastery, part of my altar-cleaning job was to arrange the objects, the flower vase, the bowl of water, and the bowl of ash for the incense stick, on the surface of the altar in front of the Buddha statue. After months of rigorous meditation practice, I found that I could move these objects slowly on the altar until I felt something like an electrical spark, and that placement would be their correct relationship to one another.

We also recognize the balance of our bodies in space. The more symmetrical we feel physically, the more comfortable we are. In fact, balance on every level is experienced as ease. As Sigmund Freud said, the organism is driven by its desire for tension release, which it recognizes as pleasure.

Another important aspect of balance for the process of evolution is our ability to recognize justice. As we begin to understand the continuity between our individual nature and all nature, the cultivation of goodness, or justice, takes on an essential, practical role in our spiritual development. The free flow of the motion of life between other people and ourselves is felt simultaneously as love and detachment, love without manipulation. If we are too passive or too aggressive, that flow is impeded. It is impossible to hurt something outside of ourselves without distorting our own nature, without limiting ourselves. In this sense, we always love our neighbor as we love ourselves.

The Sanskrit word *dharma* is translated as justice, and is also used to mean the nature of the universe, as well as the teaching of the nature of the universe. To recognize the dharma of a situation, and to respond dharmically, is to be unified (uncontrived) in our perception and our actions.

When we live in the center of our space, the center of consciousness, we perceive all aspects of life with an equal "single eye," and respond with a unified, free heart. From this perspective we can see all sides of a circumstance at once, we live in the ethical center of situations. Our response will then naturally benefit everyone involved. We are aligned with, part of, and able to witness the spontaneous unwinding of our lives toward clarity and love.

Chapter Four

DESIRE AND SPONTANEITY

Our Relationship with the Universe

There is an intrinsic link between ourselves and the vast unknown spaciousness of the universe. This link is our spiritual life, the innermost ring of the mandala, beyond or deeper than our entanglement with the world. We may recognize it first in glimpses, gazing at the night sky perhaps, or during a solitary walk on the beach—we are suddenly aware of our kinship with the elemental mystery of life. We are held, we are even nurtured, by some presence beyond the edges of our dream.

The Jewish philosopher, Martin Buber, relates a recurring dream through which he came to recognize his personal relationship with the universe. The dream always began with something happening to him. Sometimes it was a wild animal trying to tear the flesh from his arm, until he cried out.

Each time it is the same cry, inarticulate but in strict rhythm, rising and falling, swelling to a fullness which my throat could not endure were I awake, long and slow, quiet, quite slow and very long, a cry that is a song. When it ends, my heart stops beating. But then, somewhere, far away, another cry moves towards me, another which is the same, the same cry uttered or sung by another voice. Yet it is not the same cry, certainly no "echo" of my cry but rather its true rejoinder, tone for tone not repeating mine, not even in a weakened form, but corresponding to mine, answering its tones—so much so, that mine, which at first had to my own ear no sound of questioning at all, now appears as questions, as a long series of questions which now all receive a response.

Finally, he wrote, the dream took on a new form:

At first it was as usual (it was the dream with the animal), my cry died away, again my heart stood still. But then there was quiet. There came no answering call. I listened, I heard no sound. For I awaited the response from the first time; hitherto it had always surprised me, as though I had never heard it before. Awaited, it failed to come. But now something happened with me. As though I had till now had no other access from the world to sensation save that of the ear and now discovered myself as a being simply equipped with senses, both those clothed in the bodily organs and the naked senses, so I exposed myself to the distance, open to all sensation and perception. And then, not from the distance but from the air round about me, noiselessly, came the answer. Really it did not come; it was there. It had been there—so I may explain it—even before my cry: there it was, and now, when I laid myself open to it, it let itself be received by me. I received it as completely into my perception as ever I received the rejoinder in one of the earlier dreams. If I were to report with what I heard it I should have to say "with every pore of my body." As ever the rejoinder came in one of the earlier dreams, this corresponded to and answered my cry. It exceeded the earlier rejoinder in an unknown perfection which is hard to define, for it resides in the fact that it was already there.*

---

*Buber, Martin, *Between Man and Man* (New York: Macmillan Company, 1985, 2nd edition).

This is the mystery—that all of our struggle to survive and grow and understand and love, that all of our misfortunes and challenges and triumphs have all along been the unfolding of a dialogue between ourselves and our wholeness, the unbroken fundamental consciousness of the universe. This wholeness functions as a perfect parent to us—answering our questions, supplying us with circumstances which perfectly fulfill our intentions, needs and desires. Although life is still a matter of "I and thou," both the I and the thou have deepened into a new type of communion which is our primary relationship—to the universe, to God, to our own completed self.

There is, at root, no separation between our mind and the intelligence of the universe, and no separation between mind and substance. Just as the Indian guru is able to visualize a pendant and pull its material form from the air, we shape the events in our lives from the fecund clay of our mind.

* * * * *

There are two main aspects of our relationship with the universe—desire and spontaneity. Desire is the motivation for all circumstances in our lives. Spontaneity is the automatic unfolding of circumstances as a result of our intention.

In order to have a lucid relationship with the universe, we must know what we want. Before that, the universe is responding to our own conflicted, fragmented needs and images. Because we do not yet know our own mind, life appears arbitrary and even cruel. But our misfortunes are always part of our learning, growing process. As we progress, our desires become more unified. At some point, we begin to clearly witness the correspondence between inner and outer reality. As Goethe wrote, "The moment one definitely commits oneself, then Providence moves too; all sorts of things occur that never otherwise would have occurred." The growing communion of the fragmented consciousness with its wholeness is played out in the world of tangible events.

C.G. Jung was probably the first Western psychologist to discuss this aspect of nature, calling it "synchronicity." Jung saw an example of synchronicity in the accuracy of the *I Ching*, the Chinese book of oracles. The *I Ching* answers one's question to it with a reading selected by a throw of coins. Even the throw of coins seems to be simply a ritual, serving to strengthen the concentration of the participant. Many people have found that it is enough to have their question or problem in mind and open the book "at random" to find startlingly appropriate advice. Concentration is important in the use of an oracle because it unifies our intention, thus increasing our access to the wisdom and power of the universe.

Synchronicity functions in all aspects of our lives, from the most mundane to the most elevated. Some examples are so ordinary that they might pass for coincidences, except for the frequency with which they occur. Our car breaks down, forcing us to take the bus to work. On the bus, an old friend who has been on our mind for days is sitting across from us.

Other examples seem more strikingly related to our needs for growth or healing. A woman who has always had money suddenly finds herself completely broke. At first, she is terrified, bitter, furious. But two years later she has had the satisfaction of discovering her abilities to take care of herself in the world. Sometimes we lose the object of our desire, only to realize that we have all along had a more essential desire that can now be fulfilled. This is what happened to me when I was no longer able to dance. I was forced into a new way of life which turned out to be much more satisfying to my spiritual needs.

Desire, or intention, or vision, shapes the course of our circumstances. Eventually we can consciously use desire (or prayer) as a powerful creative tool. As long as our desires are not yet unified, however, they are not always aligned with the needs of our organism. We can therefore use this tool to maneuver ourselves into further imbalance. If, for example, we are motivated by an unfulfilled childhood desire for appreciation, now expressed as hunger for status, we may overuse a part of ourselves, such as our intellect or our physical strength. This kind of overuse can be sustained only so long before it results in injury or illness. What we see at work here is the healing mechanism of our wholeness, putting a limit on our imbalance.

We can never entirely create the course of our lives, again for the reason that we are not aware of all our needs. We can exert our creative vision on our lives only in balanced dialogue with the spontaneous unfolding of the universe. We must allow for the spontaneity of our organism's movement toward enlightenment.

In this way, creation requires reception. Creativity and receptivity are really two aspects of a single motion; like the inhale and exhale of breath, one does not operate without the other. We can only create to the extent that we allow ourselves to be created by the natural flow of circumstances in our life. Disturbance of this balance, which is present to some extent in everyone, diminishes both our perceptive functions (sensation, perception, understanding) and our creative effectiveness. Therefore, we do not create our life, nor does life create us, but we and our environment, we and our circumstances, are a single, dynamic unity.

The effectiveness of our intention, or prayer, depends on our concentration. The intensity of our concentration is the result of wholeheartedness. When our lives seem to be proceeding in a random way, when we feel futile and dissatisfied, we should examine ourselves for ambiguity in our desires. We may think that we want money, for example, and make an effort in that direction without any luck. On close examination, however, we may discover that we have much resistance to success.

It can be very helpful to use the techniques of visualization which are becoming popular today to strengthen your creative influence on your life. It is important to do the exercises in two phases. The first is the clear articulation and image of the desired circumstance. You can form a mental picture of whatever it is you want and, at the same time, repeat a verbal phrase to yourself describing the circumstance, three times. Again, this should be done with as much concentration as possible. Watch yourself carefully for conflicts, for hesitation, or any negative response to the visualization. Try to feel the intensity of your desire and to focus without distraction as you do the exercise.

The second phase is letting go of it, the complete relinquishment of the will. I equate will with desire because I believe that our desires act on the world. You can let go of your mental picture by simply watching it dissolve in your mind and becoming aware of the clear space of your consciousness. Keep breathing, smoothly and evenly. In any kind of healing or visualizing work, the benefit always occurs on the release of our effort. We must let things fall into place by themselves, or else our organism becomes more tense and fragmented and thus cut off from its relationship with the universe.

Our desires are the key to every aspect of our fulfillment. We can learn to navigate along the actual currents of our lives by recognizing and allowing ourselves to be pulled by the impulses of our deepest needs. Zen calls this "following an arrow around a tree."

Gradually the will is transmuted into a profound attunement to ourselves. Our system of attraction and repulsion, this pervasive, vital aspect of our organism, does not diminish as we evolve, but it matures. It becomes more and more refined as we grow more conscious of it. It is the thread which keeps us on course. As we fundamentally desire wholeness, we can depend on our authentic desires to lead us wherever we need to go in our progress toward that goal.

It is interesting that Sigmund Freud foreshadowed our understanding of this dimension of life when he claimed that dreams are wish fulfillments. If all life emerges from a fundamental integrative level of consciousness, then it is likely that our waking life serves the same purpose as our dream life. It cleans out, or spins out, the desire content of our buried consciousness, the thread that unfolds toward enlightenment. There is also a symbolic, "dream-like" logic to the things that happen to us, relating to our personal evolution. We can understand our circumstances in the same way we understand our dreams, as a message about our struggle for wholeness. In the last chapter, we will further explore how this applies to healing ourselves of illness.

As desire, which is always the desire for release, becomes unified, we come to a central yearning of our whole being for complete release. This is the desire for enlightenment. It is the desire to be without desire, the striving of the fragmented part for union with its full self.

* * * * *

Our growing awareness of the responsiveness of the universe is an authentic basis for faith. We begin to trust that whatever happens to us has potential value for our self-realization. The basic intelligence of the universe is more reliable than our own designs, because it responds not to our surface whims, but to our very deepest, even unconscious needs and long-obscured intentions.

We can say that faith is the ability to surrender to gravity, to release our defense against the natural motion of life. Anyone who has witnessed even a glimpse of the spontaneity of the universe knows that in order to live well, one's own will must be coupled with the willingness to surrender to circumstance.

As we mature, a shift occurs in our identification and loyalty from the matrix of our childhood to the more expanded and subtle chrysalis of the universe. I have been privileged to watch this transition in many of the people who have come to work with me.

A man of forty named Gregory struggled with his resentment toward his dominating parents. His dilemma had been resolved into a single kernel of incongruity. He recognized his potential for abiding happiness and for articulating this happiness as a skilled poet. He sensed what he called his "largeness of being." But in his childhood family he had been treated as the dumb one, the one who couldn't make it in the world, the one doomed to failure. There was a tormenting gap between what Gregory knew about himself and life and what he dared to be, how he dared to live. He was amazed at the tenacity of the bonds that held him to this destructive memory. He said it was his "lifeline;" if he let go of his family (and his role in the family), he would perish. Of course, at one time it had been true, even this poisonous lifeline had been his assurance of survival. The old terror of being unloved, unknown, uncared for was so familiar to him, it went almost unnoticed. But it guarded the threshold to the spiritual realm where he would find the freedom to live as he wanted to.

We cannot leap into freedom. Gregory's path was a slow dawning realization that the personality he had developed in the context of his family was not his essential nature. The perimeters of the world he had learned in his childhood were imaginary boundaries, a legacy of fear and ignorance.

It takes courage to give up the struggle for our parents' love, to become someone new, someone original, a person no one else entirely recognizes. It takes courage to allow our life to follow its authentic course beyond the scope of society's system of category and competition. At first we feel we will be alone, unloved and unloving, alienated from the warmth and respect of other people.

We find, however, that as we loosen our fixed relationship to the past, we are less alienated from life around us. We are no longer afraid to communicate ourselves to others. We are able to risk loving them, knowing that our own identity does not depend on their acceptance of us.

Our childhood pain, and our parents' pain which is now ours, is not only our prison, but also our path to freedom. Wherever we have been injured, our process of self-healing brings us particular self-knowledge and security. When we realize how fluid and imaginary our limitations really are, we can accept our unique path, our particular scheme of obstacles, as part of the flawless working of evolution. For most of us, life is never free of problems, but as we mature, our problems become less of a burden. We come to see them as part of our dialogue with the universe.

Most religious teachings begin with the practice of loving God as our mother and father. Our ability to love the universe as our parent depends on our earliest experience of nourishment and love. As human love is always to some extent imperfect, it is often difficult for us to accept and rely on the perfect love of the universe.

Anthropologists define religion as the extension of our filial relations to the universe. Although this perspective is somewhat limited, it contains an important truth. Most of us, even if we claim to be atheists, live with some concept of otherness from which pleasure and misfortune seem to come. This conscious or unconscious sense of a godhead serves to maintain our childhood sense of being loved or hated, betrayed or guilty, special or doomed. According to the values we have attributed to this power, we subject ourselves to an economy of pleasure and accomplishment. We feel that God wants us to be obedient, or self-effacing, or sexually repressed, or whatever it was that our parents approved of. And whatever survival patterns we developed to defend against our parents' upbringing are now directed against the education which life provides for us. By unraveling these projections to their source, we can finally recognize the true benevolence of the universe.

Our unquestioning dependence on a distant God is gradually, after many stages, transformed into an identification of our own actual nature with perfection. This process has been described in many ways. Jesus Christ is said to have expressed it as "I and my father are one." Sathya Sai Baba describes the stages of spiritual work as "First you are in the light, then the light is in you, then you and the light are the same." Meister Eckhart said, "I have given up God for his sake." And the legendary Zen master Bodhidharma, when asked to comment on the sacred truth, said, "Limitlessly open. Nothing is sacred." It has all along been our own self that we are learning to love and to trust and to become.

As I have stressed in the preceding chapters, we approach oneness with the universe while at the same time deepening our dualistic relationship with it. Therefore prayer can be as useful to our spiritual development as meditation practice. Whereas meditation develops fusion of oneself and the environment, prayer cultivates the total gathering of one's own integrity in communication with another. With practice, we may be able to detect that our relationship with the universe is even more than a dialogue of desire and fulfillment. It is an exchange of love between the fundamental atmosphere of the universe and our own heart.

It is interesting that our culture is beginning to conceive of a female Goddess. The Goddess is not only an important metaphor to express the growing self-discovery of women today. I think this development also points to a change in our religious sensibility in general. Feminist author Kim Chernin writes that God as Mother represents "a universe, fundamentally compassionate." Perhaps we have begun to sense that the universe is designed for our growth, that it is a source of nourishment and wisdom.

The worship of God as an object outside ourselves, or as an entity apart from the world, is, I believe, a beginning stage of religious practice. Devotion exercises the heart. It creates a particular kind of momentum, the release of which is bliss, needing no object. As we progress, our goal becomes self-realization ("you and the light are the same"), and loving merges with knowing. At the same time, we are always in relation to that other which is our own perfection. Thus, God is more than a metaphor. The fact that we have instructed ourselves to call it by a word, "God," and to focus on it with our fullest intensity, reflects the natural evolution of wisdom. We never entirely leave behind one stage to go on to the next; each stage is incorporated as we mature. Therefore, all religious perspectives, all of our various relationships to God, are true.

Spiritual progress appears to be a matter of emotional refinement. As understanding deepens, we still love what may be called God, but without sentimentality or hysteria. We still feel awe at the inconceivable intelligence and grandeur of the universe, but there is no longer guilt, no sense of abjectness in our relationship to it. We perceive ourselves as the expression of this grandeur, as well as its servants. Little by little, God is born in the world as the world. Then there is no longer any need to imagine a deity. All that is necessary to attain even the most enlightened condition is to carefully witness our own life.

For a growing number of people today, spirituality has taken a leap forward in shedding its old rules and limitations of imagery and metaphor. We are beginning to realize that the height of religious experience is not something outside ordinary life but the normal and inevitable quality of life itself, life unbound. A popular notion has emerged in the last few years that we are entering a new age, a new level of spiritual maturity. Perhaps what we are sensing is this greater intimacy, greater directness in our relationship with the universe. This new religious sensibility is based on our own actual attunement to spirit.

A poem by Dylan Thomas begins, "There was a Saviour, rarer than radium, crueler than truth, commoner than water," and ends, "Now in the dark, there is only yourself and myself." Thomas' message can be read as the conclusion of the age before this new age. It is the message of the existentialists. Our newly emerging spirituality is based on this message which brought both new freedom and new anxiety to the twentieth century. We are alone here, the existentialists said, there is no deity guiding us or giving our lives meaning. We alone are responsible for our destinies. There is nothing to give ourselves to or lose ourselves in, nothing above the individual self.

In this simple but earthshaking shift from the abstract to the particular, we come to a new level of contact with the bare facts of our lives, with experience itself. The existentialists left us a world in which we have neither to ask permission nor make confession for our actions. They stripped away the general, static values of traditional religion which had dulled our sensitivity to the true, spontaneous direction of our growth. In the attempt to rely entirely on the wits of the individual self, we have come to a much deeper understanding of what that self is.

Science, too, has been busy in this century attempting to find the essential structure of life. Science has "unlocked" matter, discovering that matter is bound energy. Now it is trying to unlock energy, to find its basic components. I think that within energy they will eventually find consciousness.

But in touching consciousness, we touch a realm beyond manipulation. We come to the source of creation, which perhaps we can understand, but which we will probably not be able to transform. More likely, its discovery will transform us. We may find that consciousness is irreducible; it is the bottom nature of the visible world. Consciousness is not something that can be analyzed or reproduced, but a potential, a basic fecundity. Only human beings are capable of becoming aware of this basic dimension of our mind, which is also the mind of the universe. If we want to proceed in our understanding of the universe, we must advance in our knowledge of ourselves.

But understanding the self cannot be accomplished by the usual analytical methods of science. Scientists are even attempting to artificially create a self. I do not think they will succeed. In order to create an intelligence comparable to human intelligence, they must invent a machine capable of attaining enlightenment, which every human being has the capacity for. They must create a machine which is in the process of evolving toward omniscience.

At a lecture several years ago, the physicist Heinz Pagels related an anecdote from his encounter with the Tibetan Dalai Lama, the spiritual and political leader of Tibet. The Dalai Lama had said that he believes in reincarnation. Dr. Pagels asked, "If we create a human being through artificial intelligence, will that be a reincarnate being?" The Dalai Lama's response was, "When you place this being in front of me, we will have this conversation again."

* * * * *

It is the paradox of human life that we are entirely alone, entirely responsible for our own selves, and also inextricably unified with the whole of nature. The existentialists said that we must exert our own order, our own creativity on a random universe. Now many of us are finding that our creativity is part of the order of the universe. This universe is inseparable from our own mind, our own creativity. It is a very different place than the alien, barren, random environment perceived by the existentialist "Everyman" who suffers incurably from the "human condition." It is "a universe, fundamentally compassionate." It is, as Trungpa Rinpoche said, "a world full of trustworthy emptiness." It mirrors our basic, tenacious love for ourselves. Samuel Beckett has one of his characters in "Endgame" say, "You're on Earth, there's no cure for that." Now it seems that being on Earth may be all the cure we need.

We need not create our own meaning in this universe. The spontaneous motion of life toward unity is meaning in itself. The pain stuck in our bodies is stagnant meaning, which simply needs breath and awareness to move again. The meaning of life, the clear light of love and wisdom, rides through our body on our breath, more deeply and tangibly as we evolve.

Chapter Five

MEDITATION

A monk said to Zen Master Nansen, "Seng Chao said, 'The whole universe is of one and the same root as my own self, and all things are one with me.' This I find very hard to understand." In reply, Master Nansen pointed to a flower blooming in the courtyard and said, "Most people see this flower as if they were in a dream."

The purpose of meditation is to realize our unity with the fundamental, unbroken ground of life. Meditation is basically the practice of quieting the mind on deeper and deeper levels until we reach the underlying, subtle consciousness that is the root of all things. But a quiet mind does not mean the absence of thoughts. It means a mind that does not interfere with or distort the natural flow of sensations, feelings, perceptions, images, and thoughts through the open field of our consciousness. A quiet mind is clear space, what the Buddhists describe as a primal state of pure presence. It is a mirror for the entire experience of inner and outer life.

A quiet mind is an undistracted mind. Although we may be fully, passionately involved in whatever is occurring, we remain grounded in the awareness of our fundamental space-consciousness. We thus experience life directly and thoroughly, stripped of the dream of our own projections.

Buddhist tradition says that the human being has three levels: body, speech and mind. As I explained in Chapter Three, this triad can also be described as sensation, emotion and awareness. The level of speech, or emotion, includes our breath and energy system, which is the mediation between our body and mind. As we practice meditation, our breath becomes increasingly fine and subtle, until both breath and awareness permeate our body. This unifies the three levels of body, speech and mind. As the mind is unified with the body, it becomes balanced and tranquil. Zen Master Shunryu Suzuki said, "To stop your mind does not mean to stop the activities of the mind. It means your mind pervades your whole body."

Most of us shift our mind slightly every time we breathe. As we progress in meditation, we are gradually able to sit still, quiet the mind, and breathe all at the same time. Our breath passes smoothly and freely through the clear space of our consciousness. We are able to feel and think without disturbing the balance of our mind and body.

The calmer we become, the more deeply we feel the motion of energy and breath passing through us. This motion is a spinning out of the inertia (repression) in our body. With each breath more territory, more inner space, is reached. Our sensation of ourselves expands and intensifies. The breath penetrates our bound emotion, bringing old feelings and memories to awareness. Thus we gradually attain a self-knowledge which is both an understanding of our history and an awakening of consciousness throughout our organism.

One form of Zen meditation is called Shikan-taza. It is a practice of sitting without any object of concentration. It is taught that just sitting is all that is necessary for the attainment of complete enlightenment. Undisturbed, the spontaneous integrating of breath, mind and body will unravel all the densities of unconscious life.

Buddhist teachers caution their students not to forcibly hold the mind still. They say that a quiet mind is a "non-abiding" mind. If we allow our thoughts to arise and dissolve without getting involved in them, they gradually subside. If we hold our mind still, we make more tension and inertia instead of less. Many people misunderstand this teaching and attempt to make themselves mentally dull and unresponsive. Actually, the exercise of allowing the mind to function without interference or elaboration increases both the concentration and fluidity of our mental capacity. Our habitual surface thoughts give way, making new levels of cognition accessible.

Much of the process of quieting the mind consists of listening to its persistent noisiness. At first, this listening should be done with care. Although our thoughts are usually the most petty trivia (the author speaks for herself), they cannot be considered unimportant. It is these small concerns which make up our general attitude toward life, even affecting the unfolding of our life circumstances. We should become aware—are our thoughts usually anxious, angry, grieving? This alertness to the mind is in itself the beginning of the lucid emptiness of undistracted meditation.

Our habitual thought patterns are also important in another way. They are signals from repressed emotions burdening and constricting our mind and body. Most of us are not aware how much time we spend fighting with people in our mind, grieving for past love, or thinking of plans to insure our survival in some way. Once we acknowledge these communications, we have tapped the hidden life in ourselves and we can allow our breath and consciousness to disperse our bound energy.

Meditation gives us a deeper perspective on life. We cease identifying with only parts of ourselves, like our physical appearance or our feelings (anger, grief, etc.). We begin to see that these parts are dynamic processes, capable of change. The witnessing of our thoughts in meditation prepares us to witness all of our life with the same non-abiding quality. As we learn not to like some thoughts and dislike others, but to allow all our thoughts to pass through us with fluidity, we find that we are able to accept "outer" circumstances with the same equanimity. When the mind does not get stuck anywhere, when it neither censors nor exalts, our perception of situations becomes more even. We begin to get the whole picture.

As the space of our mind opens and expands, time slows down, moments seem longer. Time and space are inseparable. As we let go of our grip on space (our mind), we let go of our grip of time. This produces, and reflects, a profound change in our attitude toward living. We are able to allow time to pass, which means we are able to allow ourselves to rest. As is taught in Western religion, rest is a necessary component of the creation of the world. Because of our emphasis on control, and our fear of letting go and doing nothing, many of us are damaging our health and the health of the planet. Witnessing ourselves in meditation engenders a deep appreciation and trust for the working of nature, our basic harmony and intelligence. We see that it is crucial to allow this intelligence to function freely. Just as our bodily organs are hindered by tension and overwork, our natural process of spiritual evolution functions best when we are relaxed.

At the core of the meditation experience is the paradox of being and nothingness. Although the sensation in meditation is one of continuous dissolving in space, or surrendering to the spontaneous unfolding of consciousness, there is at the same time an intensely felt sense of existing, of becoming real.

As we become ourselves, the power of our being literally breaks out of its constricting shell. What begins as a vague yearning for peace or for freedom is later felt as a surging river, pushing its way into all the numb areas of our body and mind.

This movement is the great driving power of symmetry, dissolving our entanglement, making us whole.

We begin to inhabit ourselves through and through. It has often been said that the body is the temple. In meditation, we know what it means to sit in our temple. It is interesting that the Eastern concept of undistorted consciousness has a counterpart in the Jewish teaching that there should be no images in the temple. As we rid ourselves of images, projections of fantasy onto ourselves and the world around us, our whole body awakens to the present. We learn to live right in the center of our space, receiving and affecting the world with an accuracy not possible from a more limited perspective.

Meditation helps us to develop self-reliance. Our inner monologue usually reflects our obsession with the circumstances of our life. As our mind becomes quiet, we achieve a degree of independence from these circumstances. Although most of us try to fill our lives with things which bring us pleasure, such as family, professional accomplishment, or various forms of entertainment, none of these things bring lasting happiness unless we are also happy independently of them. Happiness is the basic sensation of being alive, and the work of meditation is to penetrate whatever is blocking that sensation. Once I heard a yogic master asked to define happiness. He said, "Happiness is a matter of the way one breathes."

Meditation develops freedom from habit. We have a tendency to define ourselves by limited ideas of identity, such as "I am a good person" or "I am an artist." Although we use these self-images to understand and explain ourselves, when they are rigidly maintained they limit our potential for growth and change. They become static mental constructions, blocking the free flow of life through the open space of consciousness. Our actual being is something more primary than any definition we can make of ourselves. This is how the famous ninth-century Chinese Zen Master Rinzai described it:

> O Brethren, the Mind-Reality has no definite form. It permeates and runs through the whole universe. In the eye it acts as sight; in the ear it acts as hearing; in the nose it acts as the sense of smell; in the mouth it speaks; in the hand it grasps; in the foot it walks. All these activities are originally nothing but one single Spiritual Illumination, which diversifies itself into harmonious correspondences. It is because the Mind has in this way no definite form of its own that it can so freely act in every form.

Rigid forms are sustained by habit, or inertia. As the teaching of Castaneda's Don Juan illustrates, the only thing keeping us from becoming a crow, or whatever shape we might desire, is our strong conviction that we are bound to whatever form we currently have. Basically our identity is consciousness itself, and thus our creativity is ultimately unlimited. The significance of this for those of us who are not spiritual masters is that we have at least more flexibility than we usually recognize. We need not fear annihilation if we loosen our attachment to familiar ways of seeing ourselves, if we let our lives change and move on. If Don Juan can so thoroughly conceive of himself as a crow, then surely we can conceive of our own lives without addiction, despair, illness.

Meditation gives a sense of actuality to spiritual work. There is nothing theoretical about feeling oneself come alive, cell by cell, in the simple act of sitting and breathing.

The first meditation taught in Zen is usually the counting of breaths. The student counts every inhale or every exhale from one to ten, over and over. Sometimes it is taught that you must return to one again, wherever you are in the count, every time you have a thought. Although eventually we do not want to force the mind into silence, this practice helps the beginner to become acutely aware of his or her mental process. Once you have gained some steadiness in your awareness of yourself, you may proceed with the count, allowing your thoughts to come and go naturally. You need only return to one if you find that you have become so immersed in your thoughts that you have actually stopped counting.

For most of us, fascination with the content of our thoughts dies hard. We find repeatedly that we have given up the count to follow through on some internal scene. We must try to convince ourselves that this spectacle of our mind is all just the sub-plot of our lives. The main theme is the steady deepening and expanding of consciousness. As we persist, we find that our mind does very gradually accumulate concentration. I say accumulate because the quality of our attention becomes an almost tangible presence, with weight and stability.

Trying not to think in beginning meditation serves another purpose as well. It changes the habitual relationship between the levels of mind, breath and body. Our tape loops of mental chatter constantly reinforce our patterns of repression. If we are able to refrain from them, even for a moment, those patterns are loosened. The many techniques for focusing the mind are all meant to distract us from our habitual patterns so that our natural motion toward balance can function. Eventually, though, the object of focus must also be released.

One such focusing exercise is to carefully watch your breath, without trying to manipulate it in any way. After some time, as the body and mind become more relaxed and open, the breath will of itself slow down and become smoother and easier.

You can also choose a simple object to visualize, such as a flame, a rose, or a geometrical shape. It is usually taught to picture the object in your forehead between and slightly above your eyebrows. It is important to hold the image steady as you breathe smoothly and evenly. Objects can also be visualized in other parts of the body, for example, along the spine to open the energy system, as I will describe in the last chapter.

Another method of focusing attention is the use of mantra, the repetition of some sound or phrase, to the exclusion of all other thoughts. Traditional meditation sounds from Eastern practices serve not only to focus the mind but also to open and balance the body-mind with their particular vibration.

To understand why certain sounds can be used to evolve (free) our consciousness, we have to return to the mirror-like nature of our body-mind anatomy. Every part of ourselves reflects the vibrational pattern of our whole organism. To stimulate our vocal apparatus stimulates the whole body, and to stimulate a part of that apparatus with specific sounds stimulates the corresponding part of the body. The Hindus possess an ancient system of sounds for stimulating and opening the different energy centers of the body. For example, they use the sound "lung" for opening the bottom chakra located at the base of the spine. You can try repeating this sound yourself and see if you can feel how this sound reaches that part of your body. They use the sound "hung," the same syllable with a different consonant, to open the throat chakra.

Because of the mirroring effect, any repression in our body is also reflected in the vocal apparatus. Our throat and mouth will always be to some extent constricted and asymmetrical (depending on the shape of our consciousness). Besides, any direct stifling of vocal self-expression, be it speech, creativity, anger, tears, cries for help, etc., affects our vocal anatomy and the quality of the sound produced. Probably few human beings make it to adulthood without some specific vocal repression. Vibrational stimulation, through the use of mantra, will help loosen this repression, thus expanding and balancing our consciousness.

Once some sensitivity is gained, attention can be given to the evenness of the vocal stimulation. In our constricted anatomy, the sound will always be made more to the right or left of the mouth and throat, stimulating the body in an asymmetrical way. But with concentration, we can use the sound to correct this imbalance. Here again, we make use of our innate sense, or feel, of symmetry. We can either focus on directing the sound right through the center of our throat and mouth, or on resonating the space around the body in all directions evenly. By balancing the sound, we are balancing our awareness.

It is easiest to begin by mentally locating the center of the throat. You can find this point by making any sound and feeling where it originates.

Now breathe in and out while holding your attention at the center of your throat.

Now add the mantra to your breath.

Eventually the mantra, whether it is voiced or unvoiced, should pervade your whole being. You should feel that it is dissolving and replacing your sense of yourself. You become the mantra.

A mantra that is often used in Hindu practice is "so-hum." It is usually repeated silently. You can think the syllable "so" as you inhale and "hum" as you exhale.

Interestingly, the mantra is just as effective if unvoiced, if repeated silently without articulatory movements. The vibration of the thought will affect the body, energy and mind.

In a similar way, the use of mental imagery affects our whole organism. If we meditate on compassion, for example, even though it is only our idea of compassion, our heart will gradually open to its (innate) empathic concern for others.

Tibetan Buddhism has a practice in which the student visualizes him or herself as a deity in all of its physical and mental power and harmony. The student also cultivates "divine pride" while doing this visualization. Since all of our pain is a distortion, or veiling, of our perfection, our true balance can be awakened by holding some image of this perfection in our mind.

After any focusing or centering work with images or mantras, the object of the focus should be dissolved in the clear space of consciousness. We are never really centered until we can settle naturally, without any holding or willing, into the balanced condition. However, each effort at centering will allow us to settle a little closer to the ideal.

As our concentration accumulates and our mind becomes relatively balanced and calm, we can practice just sitting without any object of focus. It is important to keep your body upright in the sitting position (either in a chair or cross-legged on a cushion) and as still as possible. Make your breath very fine so that it feels as if it is half breath, half mind. If you have difficulty sitting still, you can practice bringing this fine breath in through your nose and into the center of your head (between your ears), and then out again through your nose. By touching the center of your head with your breath, you stimulate your whole central axis, which will help center you in space. It will also open your finest level of consciousness, the clear space of your mind which is both inside and outside of you. Be careful in this exercise to aim your breath like a laser beam right for the center of your head and not above the center. You will know that you have aimed correctly if you can feel your whole body from that point, including the bottom of your torso.

When your experience of space is steady you can practice witnessing everything that occurs in that space—sensations, emotions, images and thoughts. As long as you maintain your identification with clear space, there is no need to suppress anything that passes through this space. A Tibetan Buddhist teacher says, "The individual finds himself in the capacity of the mirror to reflect, and so all of these reflections are inherently pure."*

---

*Norbu, N., *The Cycle of Day and Night* (Barrytown, New York: Station Hill Press, 1987).

As we become the witness to life, we dissolve any limitations in our participation with it. We become a single, unbroken mirror for both subject and object, as life passes through us "leaving no trace." Yet, the more fully we identify with our fundamental space-consciousness, the more fully we inhabit our physical body. Here is the same paradox again: autonomy within oneself and fusion with one's environment grow simultaneously.

All aspects of our nature emerge from and touch the innermost core of consciousness. Whatever activity we do, if done with our full attention, our whole body and mind, will bring us closer to unity and freedom. Sexual union, love of the universe, acute metaphysical understanding, have all been said to facilitate self-realization. There are many descriptions in Buddhist literature of people attaining enlightenment on hearing a sound (completely), or seeing something with a sudden totality of vision. The Buddha himself is reported to have reached complete enlightenment when, after sitting for many days absorbed in meditation, he opened his eyes and saw the morning star.

Chapter Six

SEXUALITY

One of the great advancements of this century in the West has been the recognition of sexuality as an important aspect of emotional and mental maturity, worthy of our serious attention and healing. Sexuality has come to be regarded as a healthy, necessary part of life. This acceptance of our physical nature is a radical change from the repressive attitude of the nineteenth century which viewed sexuality as a base, almost sub-human activity.

At the same time our spirituality has also evolved. Many of us are discovering that spirituality is the essence of our humanness, rather than something "supernatural" or more than human. We have begun to accept both our spirituality and our sexuality as intrinsic to our human experience. This means that we do not have to subdue or alter our nature in order to develop our spirituality. We have to fully become ourselves.

As we have seen, the human form is designed to contain physiological, emotional, mental and spiritual life. These dimensions of life are entirely interwoven and interdependent. Nothing occurs in one aspect of ourselves without affecting all the others. If we therefore suppress one aspect of our functioning, such as our sexuality, we diminish ourselves in every way.

Sexual energy emanates from our central axis, as do all the other levels of our experience. It is an inseparable component of the essential flame of being. We can say that orgasm is the freedom of the body, just as love (or bliss) is the freedom of the heart and clarity is the freedom of the mind. But such a division is only schematic. Body, heart and mind all emerge from and lead to the fundamental unity of our being. Thus sexuality can be used as a path toward enlightenment, just as the refinement of the heart or mind. One of the most advanced forms of Tibetan Buddhism, Highest Tantric Yoga, teaches a practice of sexual union with a real or imagined partner to complete the practitioner's release into the "clear light of bliss."

Just as plants grow upward as their roots drop downward, human beings grow toward the highest, finest vibrations of our energy system as we become conscious of our sexuality and our affinity with the Earth. As we enter the spiritual dimension of life there is also a downward motion toward ground and flesh and form. Pretending not to be sexual beings, ignoring the body in this sense, creates a fragmentation in our consciousness that is mirrored throughout our entire organism.

Along with current changes in our attitude toward sexuality and spirituality in our culture, there has been a rebalancing of the relationship between women and men. Both women and men are finding that their lives are now markedly different from their parents' in the range of experience available to them.

This rebalancing, as it manifests both within society as a whole and within the individual personality, is necessary for our personal and collective evolution. It is interesting in this context to note that the known history of religion seems to be divided into two phases. The first appears to have been primarily goddess worship, organized by priestesses, celebrating the sensual forces in nature. The second consisted of male-god religions which sought a purely mental realm beyond form and shunned sensation. Hopefully our newly emerging spiritual understand-ing is a third phase in which neither men nor women will be dominant. Full maturity is the blending of sensation and aware-ness, form and emptiness.

* * * * *

The definition of gender, what it means to be male or female, is a hotly debated subject. In my own work I have found that when we dissolve our defenses in our sexual anatomy, we expe-rience a new realm of energy and consciousness which is not only sexual but also contains the distinct quality of our partic-ular gender. Because all aspects of our organism are intercon-nected, the quality of our gender is felt in all aspects of our being. Although we can say that the fundamental ground of life has no gender, until we are completely enlightened, we embody either male or female energy, based on (or reflected in) our anatomy. However, this distinction is only a matter of quality or "flavor." It has nothing at all to do with the stereotyped char-acter traits and social roles historically attributed to women and men. In fact the more we allow ourselves the full spectrum of so-called female and male traits, the more we experience our own particular gender. This is because we are allowing ourselves to be truly who we are. If we limit our behavior to conform to conventional ideas of gender, we limit our entire organism.

For example, a man who has repressed his emotional ca-pacity because he was taught that it is "feminine" to cry, has also limited both his mental and sexual experience. He will have less actual sense of his male energy than a man who has accepted his more tender, vulnerable aspects.

For many of us, the defenses in our sexual anatomy were meant not only to suppress our sexual feelings, but also the ex-perience of gender which we associate with the false, constricting images of our culture. Not wanting to be the downtrodden female or the brute male, we have cut ourselves off from the dimension of our experience which is distinctly male or female, depriving ourselves of some of the richness of our nature. Coming to know ourselves on this level is as authentic and deepening as the discovery of our own heart or our own understanding.

Personally, I struggled for a long time with a conflict between sexuality and intelligence. I feared that, as a woman, I would either be unattractive and unlovable or overwhelmingly powerful if I allowed myself to be open in both these levels of myself at once. Through my introspective work, I discovered that a lot of the binding tension in my body was meant to hold back my physical growth into womanhood. For various reasons that were important to my survival in my early adolescence, I had attempted to maintain an image of myself as a child. I felt that I needed an initiation, a formal permission, to proceed with my growth.

I began to imagine the goddess Venus sitting facing me while I meditated. I pictured her as a beautiful, wise, calm woman who was happy for me to grow into my maturity. I breathed in the nourishment of her wholehearted wish for me. Her own happiness and calm assured me that I could take whatever I needed of her encouragement without hurting or depriving her. I knew that I had chosen the right image for my healing because my response to it was unmistakable. Tension which I had held for years relaxed and new qualities of energy flooded through my body. I felt first my aching need for this feminine support and then a sense of solitary freedom to grow into my full size, to know myself as a grown woman.

It is by now a widely accepted observation that children come into the world with rudimentary sexual feelings. At first we experience loving and sexual energies as a unified response to the environment. As we grow and continue to interact and open to life, this response becomes more and more highly charged, and a natural differentiation between the levels of our experience occurs. However, these levels (sexuality, emotion, cognition) continue to function as a dynamic unity. Thus, there will always be some amount of both sexuality and emotion in all of our encounters, unless we have had to defend ourselves in childhood by fragmenting our experience.

Our parents are for each of us our personal Adam and Eve. Our perceptions of them form the foundation of all our later data gathering and conclusions about men and women. Our relationship with them is our first initiation into the sexual aspect of life. It is not, or should not be, an actual sexual relationship, but rather a chance for the child to express developing sensations and emotions without in any way jeopardizing his or her primary needs for the parents' support, guidance and protection.

However, few parents have themselves the sexual maturity to provide the ideal conditions for the flourishing of a child's sexuality. As the child responds not just to the parents' words and actions, but is sensitive to thoughts and feelings which are often beyond the parents' awareness, any sexual confusion remaining from the parents' own childhood is transmitted to the child. Therefore most of us grow up with some expectation of difficulty in our sexual relationships. These images of the past then manifest in our adult life, and we resume the struggle we began as children to resolve our conflicts with men and women, to fulfill our driving need to love and be loved.

I remember a set of pendants that were popular when I was in junior high school. The pendants were two sides of a heart, broken in some intricate design down the middle. It was the fashion for two young lovers to each wear a matching half. As it turns out, in the grown-up world as well, one often finds the partner who possesses the "other half" of one's broken heart. For example, a woman who had a remote, ungiving father will often be drawn to a man of similar qualities in the hope that she can finally convince him (the father/lover) to express affection. Very often the man she chooses will have had a mother who was excessively demanding and smothering, and he seeks in this present relationship to convince her (the mother/lover) to give him the space to feel his autonomy. The more the woman begs for his love, the more the man feels that he is being made to give something against his will that will rob him of himself. The man then further withdraws from the woman, and the woman escalates her demand for love. This is obviously an impasse, but often the need for resolution, that is, the need to convince the partner to change and satisfy one's needs, is so deeply rooted, that the couple can no more extricate themselves from the relationship than they can proceed in it. And, in fact, if they do separate, they will very likely find themselves similarly entrenched with their next lover. For it is these same maddening, familiar figures that we are compelled to woo, again and again. The primal relationship is repeated until we can see it quite clearly, until we no longer require a repetition of the same pain to wake us to the unfulfilled needs of our childhood. We can either heal our old wounds through some therapeutic means, and then enter a very different and more satisfying relationship than our usual one, or we can work with the difficult relationship to heal both ourselves and our partner. This requires that our partner is also conscious of the entrapment of the old pattern and is willing to use the relationship as a means for his or her own growth. If these conditions are present, then a sexual-love relationship can reach the level of a spiritual practice.

* * * * *

If we view spiritual maturity as the total integration of the three major realms of experience—sensation, emotion and awareness—we can see how the long-term commitment of two people toward the resolution of the barriers between them can be of value for this work. To love wholly is enlightenment. It requires the accessibility (the consciousness) of the entire organism.

The more open we are the more we can merge vibrationally with another person. Just as we can experience ourselves as continuous with open space, we can experience ourselves as continuous with another person. In the Jewish tradition, it is said that whenever two people meet, a third being comes into existence; a new configuration of energy is born of the meeting of the two.

As I've said before, each of us has a different pattern of openness to the world which constitutes our perspective on life and our mode of communicating. By perspective I mean the types of experience we are most aware of. For example, people who are primarily attuned to their emotional level will be most aware of the emotional responses of the people around them. Their interaction with other people, both verbal and non-verbal, will be suffused with emotional content.

When there is a communication problem between two people, it is often because they are each relating from different realms of their energy system. If one person is relating emotionally and the other is relating mentally, it may be difficult for them to understand each other. It may also be difficult for them to enjoy touching each other, as vibrationally they are out of sync.

In whatever aspects two people are both open, the relationship will be relatively easy and deeply satisfying. Both will be affirmed in their talents and find in their merging with one another a haven of peacefulness, a place of rest. This kind of rest is not dull. There is tremendous pleasure and the potential for very deep stimulation in the merging of two people who are open in similar ways. In this context the phrase "falling in love" takes on a surprising accuracy. Two people capable of merging deeply can actually fall within each other, immersed in each other's consciousness.

Wherever one person is more open than another, there will be conflict and the possibility of growth. Communication between two people is always exciting energetically, and this excitement can heal our habitual patterns of repression by penetrating and dispersing the bound life in each other's vibrational field.

When a couple comes to me for counseling, I will at some point in the process have them sit facing each other and sense in what part of their bodies the energy is relatively free between them and where it is not. Where both people are fairly open, there will be an automatic exchange of energy between them. If the couple has difficulty sensing this, I ask one of them to project his or her energy, like a stream of light, from his or her pelvis, chest or head towards the matching part of the partner's body. I then ask the partner to receive this energy in the same way that we allow sunshine to enter our body when we sunbathe. The couple then takes turns projecting and receiving. This cultivates attunement and increases the intensity of their exchange. Another benefit is to give a couple a clear sense of their balance of power. If one partner is overly aggressive and the other is overly passive, this will be apparent in this exercise. The more passive partner can practice projecting and the more aggressive partner can practice letting energy in.

In another exercise, I take one of their hands in my own and ask the person to contact me through their hand. I find that even people who have never considered this kind of contact can do it once it is suggested to them. I then use my own consciousness to communicate from my hand to their's. I do this with each of the partners. I then ask them to touch each other with matching body parts, for example hand to hand, or pelvis to pelvis. I ask them to communicate with each other through the consciousness in their bodies. It is difficult to describe exactly how this is done, but the intention to do it is enough to produce the result. I may ask them to feel the life in their own body, and then let that life contact the life inside their partner's body.

Here is one more exercise for sensitive couples:

Sit facing each other, looking into each other's eyes.

Now each focus your attention (still looking into each other's eyes) on the base of your own spine, breathing smoothly and evenly. Then focus on a point in front of your sacrum, in front of your spine at the level of your navel, heart, throat and center of head (inside your head between your ears), spending a few minutes at each point. If you want, you can repeat the exercise with your eyes closed, attuning yourselves to the change in the energy flow between you as you go from point to point.

Now with your eyes open, each find the center of your own head.

From the center of your own head, find the center of your partner's head.

Now find the center of your chest, in front of your spine, at the level of your heart.

From the center of your chest, find the center of your partner's chest.

Find the center of your pelvis, in front of your sacrum.

From the center of your pelvis, find the center of your partner's pelvis.

When you find your own center and your partner's centers at the same time, you will feel an increase in the contact between you.

The purpose of all these exercises is to help increase the range and depth of the vibrational exchange between partners.

They will help integrate the communication of sexual energy with the levels of love and awareness for a more satisfying relationship.

* * * * *

The injunction against sexuality found in many spiritual traditions is meant to help people cultivate higher centers, such as love and intuition, by suppressing genital feelings. But I believe that to become truly whole, we must trust ourselves with our whole nature. Rather than confine our practice to control, we can approach the perhaps more difficult task of surrender.

The new spiritual perspective requires a more complete surrender of the defensive ego because it does not pit one aspect of ourselves against another. If love and clarity are not arbitrary qualities for human beings to define, but actual conditions in the universe, we can only attain them by giving up our manipulations and opening to the unguarded reception of life.

When spiritual practices are based on repression, they can only make us more fragmented and impede our natural unfolding toward enlightenment. Our sexuality is an aspect of our inborn hunger for fusion with life which helps motivate this process. I am not saying that we must have a sexual partner to attain our wholeness. But it is necessary that we release our repression in this aspect of ourselves and allow our sexuality to become unified with the rest of our being.

Spiritual maturity means admitting that we are human, accepting and embracing the full range of our essential humanness. There is no shame but only wisdom in the design of our bodies and our inevitable participation in the momentum of nature.

Chapter Seven

SELF-HEALING

A s I have emphasized throughout this book, our fundamental nature is wholeness. All of our suffering, both mental and physical, is created by the tension of our twisting away from this underlying reality. But every tension contains within it the momentum and the path for its release. All of our pain contains the lesson of its cause, as well as its remedy. Mental and physical symptoms are communications, like dreams from those parts of ourselves which we have twisted away from. If we attune ourselves to their message, we can heal ourselves.

Self-healing is a two-fold process. It involves both loving and understanding ourselves. In fact, self-healing is learning to love and understand ourselves. Even the most painful and supposedly incurable of illnesses offers us this opportunity. For each of us, our particular suffering defines our unique path toward wholeness.

Loving Oneself

T o heal ourselves we must become intimate with ourselves. We must take up the challenge of our pain with interest and compassion. Most of us treat ourselves the way our parents and teachers treated us when we were children. We may not take our own complaints seriously, or give ourselves enough time to experience the natural movement of our organism toward balance and health. There are conditions and standards which we feel we must meet before we "deserve" to be loved and nurtured. It is important that we become aware of these deeply ingrained attitudes. We need our own unconditional love and support if we are to expose to life again those parts of ourselves that have been defended. It was because we did not feel loved that we constricted those parts, and we will not allow them to breathe again as long as we are still hating or fearing them.

Beneath our defenses and conditioning, we each possess an instinctive loyalty and love for our own self. This intrinsic bond with ourselves is an expression of our wholeness. It is therefore our bond with all life, with reality.

Several years ago a young man named Benny came to work with me. When I first met Benny, he was full of self-hatred. He was fifty pounds overweight, his skin was broken out, and his unwashed clothes emitted a bad odor. He punctuated his speech with exaggerated expressions, caricatures of anger and shame, which transformed his sad face, every few minutes, into a gargoyle. He complained bitterly that he had no friends, that he could not keep a job, that women seemed to back away from him in disgust.

On an impulse, I suggested that he sit down in front of the mirror in my office. Quickly he reached for his angry mask but it dissolved into genuine terror. "Oh no," he said, "please, I can't." He clutched his stomach and looked at me pleadingly. I also thought that I might be asking too much too soon, but my impulse was so strong that I decided to gently insist.

He hung his head as if humbled by the enormity of this ordeal and ducked into the chair. There he squirmed, squinting sideways at himself as he tossed his head this way and that.

"What do you see?" I asked him. "Just a screw-up," he answered, "A fat, ugly guy." "Look in your eyes," I said. With great effort, he fixed his gaze on the anguished face in the mirror and sought out his eyes. "What do you see?" I asked again. As he searched his eyes for the answer to my question, his face relaxed and he sat up straight for the first time since the session began and became quite still. He seemed to be remembering something. Suddenly a look of recognition lit his gaze and the first rays of tenderness. "I look very sad," he said, his eyes filling with tears. "I look like I've had a real hard time." Benny had seen himself, and quite unexpectedly for him his response had been love. He was not an ogre, he was not a gargoyle, he was a very vulnerable man who had been through a lot. In this moment he took on his own cause, he saw through his own defenses.

The Sense of Self

Becoming aware of our primary loyalty to ourselves helps us integrate our body, energy and mind. We experience a "rooting inward" of our consciousness to the core of our body. This felt knowledge of our being is inseparable from our experience of loyalty and love for ourselves.

Our sense of ourselves develops naturally and gradually as we release our defenses. Here is an exercise to accelerate the process:

Close your eyes and try to feel your sense of yourself. If you cannot do this immediately, be patient. If you keep trying, you will be able to in a little while.

Once you can feel your sense of yourself, notice where in your body you feel it. Is it in your head, your chest, your pelvis? Now try to feel your sense of yourself in other parts of your body.

Now do the same exercise with your eyes open.

If you return to this exercise every few months during your therapy or self-healing, you will probably find that your sense of yourself has become a much clearer and more pervasive feeling.

Although it seems fairly obvious that we must love ourselves in order to heal ourselves, our culture has tended to discourage self-love. Much of our religious training in the West has taught us that we are naturally bad and must will ourselves to be good. We are to accomplish this by doing good deeds, putting the needs of others before our own, generally keeping busy and avoiding any activity that might be "self-indulgent." As one person told me, "I only let myself rest when I have worked really hard." And another, "I thought by now (she was forty-five) that all my energy would be going toward helping other people." Given this cultural background, it is difficult for us to believe that our first responsibility is to ourselves, or that our compassion for others will emerge spontaneously as we gain compassion for ourselves.

Only recently has our culture begun to question its long-held view of the psyche as fundamentally split between good and evil. Although we will never, or not for a very long time, be completely free of destructive impulses, we can understand that those impulses are the result of our distortion, or defense against, reality. In a sense, we will ourselves to be bad, to resist life, and as we relinquish this resistance, our natural goodness becomes more and more apparent. Our hatred is a distortion, a sickness of love, not something separate from it.

In the same way, there is no split between our illness and our health. Illness is a distortion, a twisting away from our fundamental health.

When we realize that our primary destiny is to become fully ourselves, we can accept any circumstance that brings us closer to that goal. Illness is part of our dialogue with our wholeness; it is part of the healing process itself. Pain naturally brings our attention to those aspects of ourselves we have wanted to ignore. Above all, pain and illness are a request for our own love and care.

Understanding Oneself

I believe that we can understand much of our physical discomfort and disease as unexpressed or unacknowledged psychological distress. The longer psychological pain is kept hidden from awareness (and the greater the intensity of the pain), the more it will affect the body, first as tension and limitation in experience, and then finally as mental and physical illness. We may even find that obvious "outside" influences on the body, such as accidents, genetic history or contagion, can be created by the needs of the communicating psyche.

As I explained in Chapter One, when we withdraw our consciousness from an area of our organism, the energy flow in that area diminishes and the fascial tissues of our physical anatomy become tense. To heal ourselves means to bring consciousness and circulation back to our defended areas. There are many ways to do this. It is most important that we take the time to attune ourselves to our own specific needs. As the mental level is the foundation of our organism, with major illnesses or structural impairments we may have to resolve the mental, symbolic level of the illness in order to achieve a lasting cure. Just as with dreams, there is no general code for deciphering the meaning of an illness. However, as we concentrate on the area that needs healing, the repressed memories and emotions will gradually emerge into our consciousness. Here is an exercise that may be helpful:

Focus your attention on the part of your body that is tense or ill. Hold your attention there, breathing smoothly and evenly, keeping your mind calm and open. You may find that the pain or tension has a central knot of density. Try to focus right into the center of this knot.

Keeping your attention steady on this point, attune to your emotional level, as was described in earlier exercises. Try to feel the emotional content of the point you are focusing on. Feel the emotional quality of your breath as you hold your attention on this point. When you feel the emotional content of the tense area, you can disperse the emotion with your mind and breath. You will feel the emotion move through your body and eventually dissipate.

As you do this, be aware of any thoughts or images that occur to you. Even if they do not make sense to you at the time, you may understand them as your healing process continues.

Since pain is caused by tension, it can best be relieved by yielding to it, by settling into it. When we settle our awareness into the tense area, the energy that has been found there is able to disperse and flow freely again within our body. Once a friend of mine who was suffering from a painful illness asked a Tibetan Buddhist teacher for advice on healing herself. He told her to send her illness out to all sentient beings. At first this seemed very difficult for her to do. She did not wish her illness on anyone else. But, trusting her teacher, she decided to try it. She practiced bringing her breath to her area of pain as she inhaled and, imagining that her pain was carried by her breath out into the world as she exhaled. After a few days, she began to feel relief from pain she had had for months. She realized that she had not given her illness to anyone else as she had feared, because as soon as the pain was dispersed and "sent out" it ceased to be pain.

Probably the most important factor in healing ourselves is our intention to get well. If our desire for health is strong, we will find that our circumstances offer us everything we need for our recovery. Any conflicts we may have in our desire for health will also become clear as we understand our illness.

I don't wish to make this sound easier than it is. We almost all resent the disruption of our lives by illness and often we do not want to hear the message of our pain. To heal thoroughly requires a life change, a change of perspective, and this takes time, more time than we may wish or expect to spend. Often we must interrupt our involvement with our work or relationships to encounter our own being more directly than we ever have before. It is only gradually that we realize the great value of this encounter.

The Chakras

No one can understand the symbolism of our illness or tension better than we ourselves, but there are some general systems of the mind-body relationship that can be useful. One is the Hindu chakra system which divides our energy spectrum into different levels or qualities of energy associated with specific types of experience. The chakras are described as vortices of energy (the word *chakra* means wheel in Sanskrit). The seven main chakras are located along the spine at the coccyx, sacral area, navel, heart, throat, center of head (or between the brows), and at the top of the head. These are the qualities which the Hindus ascribe to the different chakras:

the coccyx: our relationship with the earth, survival;
the sacral area: sexuality;
the navel: personal power, ego strength;
the heart (located at the spine next to the heart): love;
the throat: creativity, expression, dreams;
the center of the head (or between the brows): pure awareness, self-command, intuition;
the top of the head: total spiritual awakening.

The chakras function like valves in our energy system. When our energy is repressed, the valves are closed and our organism is divided. When our energy is circulating freely, the valves are open and our organism is more unified.

117

The chakras are distinct because of their particular sensi-tivity to penetration—at these points our mind can enter most easily into the deeper, subtler levels of consciousness which emanate from the core of our body-mind. The chakras can be located quite easily by their sensitive, electrical quality. To find the chakra at your coccyx, for example, bring your attention down through your torso to the coccyx (the chakras are usually reached through the front, or anterior, of the spine). Hold your attention at the coccyx, breathing evenly, until you feel an in-crease in vibration. You may also feel a sensation of expansive-ness, or warmth, or you may feel energy moving from your coccyx area to other parts of your body. These sensations will intensify the more closely you come to touching the coccyx with your mind.

Use the same procedure for finding the other chakras—bring your attention as close to the front of the spine in the area of the chakra as you can, and breathe evenly, holding your at-tention steady, until you feel an increase in vibration. You will find that as you continue to focus on the area of the chakra, the inner space of your body will become more permeable, allowing you to locate the chakra more precisely and to approach it more closely.

Holding your attention single-pointedly on a chakra will increase your energy circulation in that particular area of the body and throughout your entire organism. If you continue to concentrate on the chakra, you will gradually penetrate to the core of yourself, to the subtle, unbroken ground of your being. All of the chakras are pathways to the same one center, or source, of our existence.

As you can see from the list of qualities associated with the various chakras, the spectrum of energy is vertical, with the sub-tler qualities emanating from the top of the head, and the denser, "earthier" qualities emanating from the coccyx.

Awakening the subtler levels of our energy system is very important for self-healing, as they pervade the denser levels. The more contact we have with the subtle ground of our being, the more creative influence we have over our body, and the more open we are to the healing influence of the universe.

Here is an exercise for opening the chakras:

Visualize a triangle with the apex up at a point between your eyebrows. If it is difficult for you to picture the triangle, try drawing it in your mind in pink, in green, in yellow, or whatever color you choose. If it is easy for you to see the triangle, or when with some practice it becomes easy, you can switch to a six-pointed star. With its balance of upward and downward triangles, the six-pointed star is a particularly integrating shape for the body-mind.

Hold the image steady between your eyebrows and breathe slowly and evenly. Keep focused on this image for five or ten minutes. Then repeat the exercise with the triangle or star at the center of your throat, the center of your chest (at the level of your heart), the navel, the sacrum, and the coccyx. Try to place the visualization deep in your body, right in front of your spine at each point. As you begin to experience yourself more subtly, you can feel that you are placing the visualization within the spine instead of in front of it.

If you have an illness or injury, concentrate longest at the chakra in the area of your illness or pain. You can also place the visualization in the center of your tension, as in the exercise I described earlier.

Any traditional chart of correspondences, such as the Hindu chakra system, can only be used as a general guide to the body-mind relationship. It is not a substitute for the subtle, uncharted work of self-attunement.

Anything that impedes the circulation of our physical and energetic systems can contribute to poor health. Particularly if we are in the process of healing ourselves, it is crucial that the air we breathe and the food we eat be relatively free of pollutants. Again, taking the time to listen inwardly is the best guide to choosing the diet and climate we need.

Imagery

Every cell of our body is in a state of constant fluidity and change. In every instant, our consciousness regenerates our organism with our habitual patterns of limitation and tension. Although these limitations were once protective movements away from painful stimulation, they are now based on the projection of our childhood circumstances onto our present experience. They are our imagination, our dream that distorts reality. We have imagined ourselves with less vision, less sexuality, less ability to love. In order to heal ourselves, we must break the spell of our imagining.

Our images dissolve as soon as we recognize them as illusory, as soon as we see through them. If we genuinely knew that our true nature was whole and infinite, we would be enlightened on the spot. As Mary Baker Eddy, the founder of Christian Science, wrote, "If God were understood instead of being merely believed, this understanding would establish health."

The body is so responsive to the imagination that we can use the power of imagery to return the body to health. We can use new, healthy symbols as an antidote to the symbols of our illness. For example, if a painful dislocation of our lower back feels as though we have been cast off our "throne," perhaps by some excessive criticism or abuse we suffered as children, we can rebalance ourselves on our sacrum by imagining that we are reinstating ourselves on our throne. The image itself, if it is the correct antidote, will move our physical anatomy. We even have the ability to reconstruct an injured or diseased part of ourselves with our visual imagination. Usually this imagery must be repeated consistently, over time, to be successful. It should, however, be done gently, without effort, so that it does not add tension to the body.

When working with healing images it is most important to remember that we are working in partnership with the underlying wisdom of our wholeness. After each session of imagining, the images should be dissolved back into the clear space of unified consciousness.

Opening to Gravity

As we become more open, we more fully receive and affect the cosmos of which we are a part. Our growing communion with the universe pulls us toward health, toward balance.

Balance is our alignment with Earth's gravity. Usually we think of gravity as a force that presses against us from outside, that might knock us down if we did not resist it. However, as we are not solid objects but vibrational (gravitational) fields ourselves, Earth's gravity moves not on us, but through us.

When we open to the movement of gravity, we discover that gravity's effect on us is not one directional, not only down-ward-moving. As we learn from Tai-Chi Ch'uan, there is also an upward-moving current that intensifies as we sink our energy downward. As we settle ourselves toward the ground, as we sur-render our defenses, this motion rises upward in us, makes our body light and buoyant and pulls us toward balance. Here is an exercise to feel this for yourself:

Sit on a chair or cross-legged on the floor. Drop your weight toward the ground (without collapsing your torso). Now drop your mind to the ground. As you drop downward, there is an automatic upward-rising current. Try to attune yourself to this current.

Now do the same exercise standing. Stand for five minutes, dropping your feet to the ground and sensing the upward current flow through your body. Do not push your energy upward. If you do not feel the current at first, keep letting go and settling to the ground. Can you feel that the floor supports you? Can you feel that this upward current keeps you upright with very little effort required on your part?

Space-Consciousness

Continue with the above exercise, settling your energy downward and sensing the upward current. Now become conscious of yourself witnessing your body and your energy. Ask yourself, "Who feels the energy?" "Who asks the question?"

As you continue to search for the "who" at the core of your experience, you will find the stillness within the motion of life, the empty space through which life passes. You are finding your unified space-consciousness which pervades and reflects all of your experience.

* * * * *

We grow by a combination of intention and surrender, creativity and grace. We are both sovereign, self-generating individuals and inseparable from the one vast expanse of love and clarity which we call the universe. The energies of the universe flow through the open field of our consciousness, deepening and maturing us. Yet only our own initiative can release our defenses against the impact of each moment. What faith it takes! To let oneself feel a little more sensation, a little more love. To relax our grip. To see through life to its subtle ground of joy, pure presence, and freedom.

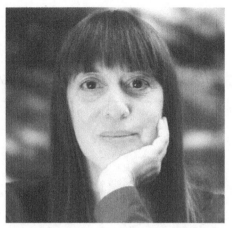

Photo by Laura Kavanau

Judith Blackstone is the founder of Realization Process, a method of integrating psychological healing, embodiment and spiritual realization. For information on Judith's books and teaching schedule, visit www.judithblackstone.com

About North Atlantic Books

North Atlantic Books (NAB) is a 501(c)(3) nonprofit publisher committed to a bold exploration of the relationships between mind, body, spirit, culture, and nature. Founded in 1974, NAB aims to nurture a holistic view of the arts, sciences, humanities, and healing. To make a donation or to learn more about our books, authors, events, and newsletter, please visit www.northatlanticbooks.com.